Chronic Kidney Disease and the Nutrition Care Process

Maureen P. McCarthy, MPH, RD, CSR, LD,

Jessie M. Pavlinac, MS, RD, CSR, LD,

and Arianna Aoun, MS, RD, CSR, LD

eat right. Academy of Nutrition and Dietetics

ISBN 978-0-88091-479-6

The views expressed in this publication are those of the authors and do not necessarily reflect policies and/or official positions of the Academy of Nutrition and Dietetics. Mention of product names in this publication does not constitute endorsement by the authors or the Academy of Nutrition and Dietetics. The Academy of Nutrition and Dietetics disclaims responsibility for the application of the information contained herein.

10 9 8 7 6 5 4 3 2

For more information on the Academy of Nutrition and Dietetics, visit: www.eatright.org

Contents

Authors and Reviewers

AUTHORS

Maureen P. McCarthy, MPH, RD, CSR, LD
Assistant Professor/Transplant Dietitian
Oregon Health & Science University
Portland, OR

Jessie M. Pavlinac, MS, RD, CSR, LD
Director, Clinical Nutrition
Oregon Health & Science University
Portland, OR

Arianna Aoun, MS, RD, CSR, LD
Clinical Dietitian, Renal
Louis Stokes Cleveland VA Medical Center
Cleveland, OH

REVIEWERS

Lori S. Brizee, MS, RD, CSP, LD
Clinical Dietitian in Private Practice
Bend, OR

Jerrilynn D. Burrowes, PhD, RD
Professor and Chair, Department of Nutrition
Long Island University Post
Brookville, NY

Sara Erickson, RD, CSR, LDN, CNSC
Pediatric Renal Dietitian
Carolinas Healthcare System (Levine Children's Hospital)
Charlotte, NC

Rachael R. Majorowicz, RD, LD
Clinical Renal Dietitian
Mayo Clinic
Rochester, MN

Jean Stover, RD, LDN
Renal Dietitian
DaVita
Conshohocken, PA

MEMBERS OF THE IDNT ADVISORY PANEL

Donna Pertel, MEd, RD
Elise Smith, MA, RD, LD

Abbreviations

AA	amino acids
ABW	adjusted body weight
ADIME	assessment, diagnosis, intervention, monitoring and evaluation (steps in the Nutrition Care Process)
AKI	acute kidney injury
Alb	albumin
ARB	angiotensin receptor blocker
A.S.P.E.N.	American Society for Parenteral and Enteral Nutrition
BEE	basal energy expenditure
BMI	body mass index
BUN	blood urea nitrogen
Ca	calcium
$CaCO_3$	calcium carbonate
CAPD	continuous ambulatory peritoneal dialysis
$Ca \times PO_4$	serum calcium–phosphorus product
CARI	Caring for Australasians with Renal Impairment
CCPD	continuous cyclic peritoneal dialysis
CfC	Conditions for Coverage (from CMS)
CHr	reticulocyte hemoglobin content
CKD	chronic kidney disease
CMS	Centers for Medicare & Medicaid Services
Cr	creatinine
CRF	chronic renal failure (replaced by CKD)
CRN	Council on Renal Nutrition
CRP	C-reactive protein
CRRT	continuous renal replacement therapy

DFO	deferoxamine
DHHS	Department of Health and Human Services
DKD	diabetic kidney disease
DM	diabetes mellitus
DPI	dietary protein intake
DRI	Dietary Reference Intake
EAL	Evidence Analysis Library (of the Academy of Nutrition and Dietetics)
EBNPG	evidence-based nutrition practice guidelines
EBPG	European Best Practice Guidelines
EDW	estimated dry weight
efBW	edema-free body weight
eGFR	estimated glomerular filtration rate
ESA	erythropoiesis-stimulating agent
ESRD	end-stage renal disease
GFR	glomerular filtration rate
GI	gastrointestinal
Glofil	glomerular filtration
HBV	high biological value
HD	hemodialysis
HDL	high-density lipoprotein
Hgb	hemoglobin
Hgb A1c	hemoglobin A1c
HTN	hypertension
IBW	ideal body weight
IDNT	International Dietetics and Nutrition Terminology
IDPN	intradialytic parenteral nutrition
IDWG	interdialytic weight gain
IG	interpretive guideline
IgA N	immunoglobulin A nephropathy
IHD	intermittent hemodialysis
iPTH	intact parathyroid hormone
IU	international unit

IV	intravenous
K	potassium
KDIGO	Kidney Disease: Improving Global Outcomes
KDOQI	Kidney Disease Outcomes Quality Initiative
LDL	low-density lipoprotein
LEE	lower-extremity edema
MAC	microalbumin-to-creatinine ratio
MBD	mineral and bone disorder
mcg	microgram
MCH	mean corpuscular hemoglobin
MCV	mean corpuscular volume
mEq	milliequivalent
Mg	magnesium
MNT	medical nutrition therapy
MUFA	monounsaturated fatty acids
MVI	multivitamin
Na	sodium
NCEP	National Cholesterol Education Program
NCP	Nutrition Care Process
NCPM	Nutrition Care Process and Model
NHANES II	National Health and Nutrition Examination Survey II
NHD	nocturnal hemodialysis
NHHD	nocturnal home hemodialysis
NHLBI	National Heart, Lung, and Blood Institute
NIDDK	National Institute of Diabetes, Digestive and Kidney Diseases
NIH	National Institutes of Health
NKDEP	National Kidney Disease Education Program
NKF	National Kidney Foundation
NLM	National Library of Medicine
nmol	nanomole

NODAT	new-onset diabetes after transplantation
nPNA	normalized protein nitrogen appearance
OTC	over-the-counter
PA	physical activity
PD	peritoneal dialysis
PES	problem, etiology, signs and symptoms
PN	parenteral nutrition
PO_4	phosphorus
POC	plan of care
PPN	peripheral parenteral nutrition
PTH	parathyroid hormone
PUFA	polyunsaturated fatty acids
RBC	red blood cell
RD	registered dietitian
RPG	Renal Practice Group
RRT	renal replacement therapy
Rx	prescription
SBW	standard body weight
SCCM	Society of Critical Care Medicine
SGA	subjective global assessment
SI	Système International d'Unités (international system of units; for scientific measurements)
TG	triglycerides
TIBC	total iron-binding capacity
TPN	total parenteral nutrition
TSAT	percent serum transferrin saturation
VLDL	very low–density lipoprotein
WBC	white blood count
WHO	World Health Organization
WNL	within normal limits

Chapter 1

Chronic Kidney Disease, Evidence-Based Practice, and the Nutrition Care Process

This guide follows the steps of the Nutrition Care Process (NCP)—nutrition assessment, nutrition diagnosis, nutrition intervention, and nutrition monitoring and evaluation—as outlined in the *International Dietetics & Nutrition Terminology (IDNT) Reference Manual* published by the Academy of Nutrition and Dietetics (also referred to as the Academy) (1). The following are also incorporated into the text, tables, and boxes in this guide:

- The Evidence-Based Nutrition Practice Guidelines (EBNPG) for Chronic Kidney Disease (CKD), which are published in the Evidence Analysis Library (EAL) of the Academy of Nutrition and Dietetics (2)
- Recommendations from publications of the National Kidney Foundation Kidney Disease Outcomes Quality Initiative (NKF-KDOQI) on nutrition (3); diabetes and CKD (4,5); CKD evaluation (6); anemia in CKD (7); hypertension and antihypertensive agents in CKD (8); and managing dyslipidemia in CKD (9)
- Recommendations from similar publications by Kidney Disease: Improving Global Outcomes (KDIGO), an international consortium of profes-

sional and patient-based organizations dedicated to kidney disease, especially its report on CKD–mineral and bone disorder (CKD-MBD) (10) and a recent update on CKD evaluation and management (11)

- Criteria for reimbursement and required documentation established by the Centers for Medicare & Medicaid Services (CMS) Conditions for Coverage (CfC) for end-stage renal disease (ESRD) facilities and CMS Medicare Part B reimbursement criteria for medical nutrition therapy (MNT) for CKD and renal transplant (12,13)
- Key points from the American Society for Parenteral and Enteral Nutrition (A.S.P.E.N.) clinical guidelines regarding nutrition support in adult acute and chronic renal failure and A.S.P.E.N. adult critical care guidelines for renal failure (14,15)
- Recommendations from the European Best Practice Guidelines (EBPG) for hemodialysis nutrition (16)
- Post–kidney transplant nutrition guidelines from the Caring for Australasians with Renal Impairment (CARI) initiative (17)

Findings and recommendations from the aforementioned sources are integrated into the chapters to which they apply—Chapter 2: Nutrition Assessment; Chapter 3: Nutrition Diagnosis; Chapter 4: Nutrition Intervention: Part 1—Planning the Nutrition Prescription; Chapter 5: Nutrition Intervention: Part 2—Implementation; and Chapter 6: Nutrition Monitoring and Evaluation.

INTRODUCTION TO CHRONIC KIDNEY DISEASE

In 2002, NKF-KDOQI published a system for classifying the five original stages of CKD (see Table 1.1) (6).

Table 1.1	Stages of Chronic Kidney Disease (CKD)
Stages of CKD	*Glomerular Filtration Rate (GFR)*
Stage 1	≥ 90 mL/min/1.73 m^2 with kidney damage
Stage 2	60–89 mL/min/1.73 m^2
Stage 3	30–59 mL/min/1.73 m^2
Stage 4	15–29 mL/min/1.73 m^2
Stage 5 and Stage 5D (D = Dialysis)	<15 mL/min/1.73 m^2

Source: Reprinted from reference 6: National Kidney Foundation. KDOQI clinical practice guidelines for chronic kidney disease: evaluation, classification, and stratification. *Am J Kidney Dis.* 2002;39(suppl 1):S1–S266. www.kidney.org/professionals/KDOQI/guidelines_ckd/p4_class_g1.htm. Reprinted with permission from National Kidney Foundation, Inc.

The KDIGO 2012 Clinical Practice Guidelines for the Evaluation and Management of Chronic Kidney Disease maintained the glomerular filtration rate (GFR) ranges for stage 1 through stage 5 CKD but split stage 3 into two categories (11).

- Stage 3a is defined by a GFR range of 45 to 59 mL/min/1.73m^2.
- Stage 3b is defined by a GFR range of 30 to 44 mL/min/1.73m^2.

Post–kidney transplant patients/clients have varying levels of renal function. Their level of CKD should be determined based on the individual's estimated glomerular filtration rate (eGFR) with MNT applied accordingly.

MNT is an essential intervention to promote ideal health parameters. Patients/clients with various health conditions and illnesses can improve their health and quality of life when they are educated on and adhere to MNT recommendations. During MNT interventions, registered dietitians (RDs) educate and counsel patients/clients on behavioral and lifestyle changes essential to encourage positive lifelong eating habits and health measures. Box 1.1 illustrates how MNT relates to the steps of the NCP (18).

Box 1.1   Medical Nutrition Therapy (MNT) and the Nutrition Care Process (NCP)

In the context of the NCP, providing MNT requires:
- Performing a comprehensive nutrition assessment (A)
- Determining the nutrition diagnosis (D)
- Planning and implementing a nutrition intervention (I) using evidence-based nutrition practice guidelines
- Monitoring (M) an individual's progress over subsequent visits with the registered dietitian (RD)
- Evaluating (E) an individual's progress over subsequent visits with the RD

Source: Data are from reference 18.

This guide focuses on the appropriate MNT for CKD stages 3 to 5D, including renal transplant. Acute kidney injury (AKI) is not addressed. The focus of MNT depends on the stage of CKD and the patient-/client-associated medical history as well as whether the encounter is an initial or follow-up visit. For instance, MNT provided for a patient/client with stage 5 CKD and diabetes who has elevated potassium and phosphorus levels but an Hgb A1c of 6.8% would be different from MNT for a stage 3a CKD patient/client with normal potassium and phosphorus levels but an Hgb A1c of 9%. Nutrition prescriptions and nutrition interventions are discussed further in Chapters 4 and 5.

Medicare Part B reimburses MNT provided by an RD or other qualified nutrition professional for patients/clients whose GFR is between 13 and 50 mL/min/1.73m² (pre-dialysis). Post–kidney transplant patients/clients with any level of allograft function are covered by Medicare Part B for up to 3 years with a physician referral (19). More information can be found at the CMS Web site (www.cms.gov) by searching for "MNT." See Table 1.2 for a summary of Medicare Part B coverage for MNT (13,19).

Table 1.2   Medicare Part B Reimbursement for Medical Nutrition Therapy (MNT) for Patients/Clients with eGFR 13–50 mL/min/1.73m² and for Posttransplant Patients/Clients

Timeline	MNT Units Reimbursed	Total Hours per Year
1st year	12	3
Each subsequent year	8	2

Source: Data are from references 13 and 19.

Based on medical necessity, additional hours of MNT may be covered if the treating physician orders them due to a change in medical condition, diagnosis, or treatment regimen (13). For the first 3 years after a transplant, MNT is a Medicare Part B benefit regardless of GFR. After that time period, however, only those posttransplant patients/clients with an eGFR between 13 and 50 mL/min/1.73m² and a physician referral are eligible for Medicare Part B reimbursement for MNT.

SCREENING AND REFERRAL FOR MEDICAL NUTRITION THERAPY ENCOUNTERS

The Academy's EBNPG for CKD (2) recommend the following practices for screening and referral of patients/clients with CKD:

- MNT should be provided by the RD for individuals with CKD because "MNT prevents and treats protein-energy malnutrition and mineral and electrolyte disorders and minimizes the impact of other comorbidities on the progression of kidney disease (eg, diabetes, obesity, hypertension, and disorders of lipid metabolism)."

- MNT "should be initiated at diagnosis of CKD, in order to maintain adequate nutritional status, prevent disease progression, and delay renal replacement therapy (RRT) . . . or transplant. MNT should be initiated at least 12 months prior to the anticipation of RRT."

- "The RD should monitor the nutritional status of individuals with CKD every 1 to 3 months and more frequently if there is inadequate nutrient intake, protein-energy malnutrition, mineral and electrolyte disorders, or the presence of an illness that may worsen nutritional status, as these are predictive of increased mortality risk."

MEDICAL NUTRITION THERAPY BASED ON THE STAGE OF CHRONIC KIDNEY DISEASE

The RD evaluates the stage of CKD and prioritizes the strategy for MNT based on nutrition issues that arise during that stage of CKD. Additionally, the RD assesses the patient's/client's level of interest in learning about his or her stage of CKD and the available social support, and, on that basis, tailors MNT education and counseling. MNT for post–kidney transplant patients/clients should be based on posttransplant renal function, which may decline over time.

Stage 3 Chronic Kidney Disease and Renal Transplant

In clinical practice, evidence-based guidelines for MNT should be applied as appropriate based on a review of the patient's/client's medical history (eg, diabetes, hypertension, lipid disorders, or obesity), stage of CKD (including kidney transplant), nutritional status, and any mineral or electrolyte imbalances. The RD should plan to coordinate care of the CKD patient/client with the interdisciplinary team to maximize the individual's care (2,12).

Stage 4 Chronic Kidney Disease and Renal Transplant

Because stage 4 CKD is defined by an eGFR of 15 to 29 mL/min/1.73m^2, MNT for CKD and posttransplant patients/clients in this stage is covered by Medicare Part B (6,11,13). As in earlier stages of CKD, MNT is based on a thorough assessment and includes coordination of care.

Stage 5 CKD, not on Dialysis, and Renal Transplant

Stage 5 CKD, not on dialysis, is defined by an eGFR of less than 15 mL/min/1.73m^2 (6,11). Medicare Part B provides MNT coverage only for patients/clients with an eGFR of 13 mL/min/1.73m^2 or greater within stage 5 CKD or for posttransplant patients/clients with this level of renal function (13). As in earlier stages of CKD, MNT is based on a thorough assessment and includes coordination of care.

Stage 5D—Hemodialysis and Peritoneal Dialysis

Stage 5D CKD, also known as ESRD, is defined by the initiation of RRT (either hemodialysis [HD] or peritoneal dialysis [PD]) (8). According to NKF-KDOQI nutrition guidelines, nutritional status should be evaluated using a combination of measures, such as protein and energy intake, body composition, and functional status (3).

CMS has released CfC for ESRD, which outline the
mandatory nutrition care plan and documentation to be
completed for each dialysis patient/client (12). Box 1.2
summarizes the CfC and corresponding interpretive
guidelines (IGs) that relate to the four steps of the NCP
(20,21). Interpretive guidelines are published by govern-
ment agencies such as CMS to guide surveyors who are
applying standards such as the CfC in the field.

**Box 1.2   Medicare Conditions for Coverage (CfC) Mandates
            Related to the Nutrition Care Process (NCP) and
            Documentation**

Nutrition Assessment
- CfC§494.80 describes requirements for patient/client
  assessment.
- Interpretative guideline (IG) tags V500-515 describe infor-
  mation to be included in assessments.
  ◦ V509 is specific to nutrition.
  ◦ Topics discussed in other tags, such as factors associated
    with renal bone disease, also relate to nutrition and may
    be completely or partially addressed by the nephrology
    dietitian in accordance with accepted practice patterns at a
    given end-stage renal disease (ESRD) facility.

Nutrition Diagnosis
- Not mandated by the Centers for Medicare & Medicaid
  Services (CMS) but a vital component of what the registered
  dietitian (RD) does.
- Should be included in documentation of nutrition care.

(continued)

Box 1.2   Medicare Conditions for Coverage (CfC) Mandates Related to the Nutrition Care Process (NCP) and Documentation (continued)

Nutrition Intervention (Including Care Plan) and Nutrition Monitoring and Evaluation
- CfC§494.90 states that an interdisciplinary team must develop and implement a comprehensive plan of care (POC) that describes services needed (ie, interventions) and outcomes (ie, monitoring and evaluation step of NCP).
- IG Tag 545 sets expectations for an outcome-oriented POC related to nutritional status.

Source: Data are from reference 20.

Chapter 2

Nutrition Assessment

Throughout the remaining chapters of this guide, a case-study approach will be used to illustrate the management of chronic kidney disease (CKD). The case study is presented in installments at the end of each chapter, adding details pertinent to the Nutrition Care Process (NCP) step discussed in that chapter.

The process of nutrition assessment includes obtaining, verifying, and interpreting data to identify a nutrition problem or diagnosis. Nutrition assessment is ongoing and involves comparing the patient's/client's data parameters to standards or expected values for his or her overall condition (1). Nutrition assessment for patients/clients with CKD requires an understanding of kidney physiology, the nutritional ramifications in the various stages of CKD, and how medical management (including medications) affects the nutritional status of the patient/client. This chapter discusses the five domains of nutrition assessment as they relate to patients/clients with CKD:

- Food- and nutrition-related history
- Anthropometric measurements
- Biochemical data, medical tests, and procedures
- Nutrition-focused physical findings
- Client history

The terminology used is from the fourth edition of the *International Dietetics & Nutrition Terminology (IDNT) Reference Manual.* Comparative standards for CKD for energy, micro- and macronutrients, fluid needs, and weight recommendations are included in this guide (1).

FOOD- AND NUTRITION-RELATED HISTORY

The food- and nutrition-related data needed to perform an assessment of a CKD patient/client include the following (1,2,22):

- Current energy and protein intake
- Fat intake
- Mineral intake (sodium, potassium, phosphorus, and calcium) from food and supplements
- Vitamin intake from food and supplements
- Fluid/beverage intake
- Fiber intake
- Caffeine intake (pertinent for hypertension and in patients/clients with polycystic kidney disease)
- The amount and distribution of carbohydrate intake for patients/clients with diabetes

Other appropriate patient-/client-specific assessment data might include enteral nutrition (including oral nutritional supplements) intake, parenteral nutrition intake, alcohol intake, and intake of bioactive substances (eg, plant sterol and/or stanol esters, soy protein, psyllium, or food additives).

The current diet prescription or pattern that the patient/ client follows, previous nutrition counseling/education, beliefs and attitudes around food, and food and nutrition knowledge regarding the protein, sodium, potassium, and phosphorus content of foods will serve as the basis for developing a CKD-appropriate diet prescription and education plan. The availability of food, the ability to prepare foods, and the eligibility and need for food/nutrition programs will also influence the care plan. The diet prescription must be developed based on the stage of kidney disease and other comorbid conditions, if any. Specific guidelines for the diet prescription are described in Chapter 4.

Medication history and current medication usage, including alternative therapies, significantly affect the nutrition assessment and diet prescription of the patient/client with CKD. Common classes of drugs used in these patients/clients include antihypertensives, phosphate binders, cardiac medications, and hypoglycemic medications. Assessment of medications should include their phosphorus and potassium content (particularly of over-the-counter products and dietary supplements); the effect of the medication(s) on the kidneys with regard to sodium, potassium, and fluid elimination; the composition of the phosphate binders, and the impact of the medications on bone health and soft tissue calcification. Boxes 2.1 through 2.5 provide information about common medications used by individuals with CKD (4,5,10,23–25).

Box 2.1   Antihypertensive Medications Used by Patients/Clients with Chronic Kidney Disease (CKD)

Thiazides
- Examples: chlorothiazide (Diuril), hydrochlorothiazide (Microzide, HydroDiuril), indamapide (Lozol), metolazone (Mykrox), metolazone (Zaroxolyn), polythiazide (Renese)
- Adverse effect relevant to CKD: Decreased serum potassium

(continued)

**Box 2.1   Antihypertensive Medications Used by Patients/
Clients with Chronic Kidney Disease (CKD)** (continued)

Loop Diuretics
- Examples: bumetanide (Bumex), furosemide (Lasix), torsemide (Dyrenium)
- Adverse effect relevant to CKD: Decreased serum potassium

Potassium-Sparing Medications
- Examples: amiloride (Midamor), triamterene (Dyrenium)
- Adverse effect relevant to CKD: Increased serum potassium

Aldosterone Receptor Blockers
- Examples: eplerenone (Inspra), spironolactone (Aldactone)
- Adverse effect relevant to CKD: Increased serum potassium

Beta-Blockers
- Examples: atenolol (Tenormin), betaxolol (Kerlone), bisoprolol (Zebeta), metoprolol (Lopressor), metoprolol extended release (Toprol XL), nadolol (Corgard), propranolol (Inderal), propranolol long-acting (Inderal LA), timolol (Blocadren)
- Adverse effects relevant to CKD: Constipation, nausea, edema

Beta-Blockers with Intrinsic Sympathomimetic Activity
- Examples: acebutolol (Sectral), penbutolol (Levatol)
- Adverse effects relevant to CKD: N/A

Combined Alpha- and Beta-Blockers
- Examples: carvedilol (Coreg), labetalol (Normodyne, Trandate)
- Adverse effects relevant to CKD: N/A

ACE Inhibitors
- Examples: benazepril (Lotensin), catopril (Capoten), enalapril (Vasotec), fosinopril (Monopril), lisinopril (Prinivil, Zestril), moexipril (Univasc), perindopril (Aceon), quinapril (Accupril), ramipril (Altace), trandolapril (Mavik)
- Adverse effects relevant to CKD: Increased serum potassium, metallic or salty taste

(continued)

**Box 2.1   Antihypertensive Medications Used by Patients/
Clients with Chronic Kidney Disease (CKD)** (continued)

Angiotensin II Antagonists (ARBs)
- Examples: candesartan (Atacand), eprosartan (Teveten), irbesartan (Avapro), losartan (Cozaar), olmesartan (Benicar), telmisartan (Micardis), valsartan (Diovan)
- Adverse effects relevant to CKD: Increased serum potassium, salty or metallic taste, nausea, diarrhea, dyspepsia

Calcium Channel Blockers: Non-dihydropyridines
- Examples: diltiazem extended-release (Cardizem CD, Dilacor XR, Tiazac, Cardizem LA), verapamil immediate release (Calan, Isoptin), verapamil long-acting (Calan SR, Isoptin SR), verapamil-COER (Covera HS, Verelan PM)
- Adverse effects relevant to CKD: Constipation, nausea, edema

Calcium Channel Blockers: Dihydropyridines
- Examples: amlodipine (Norvasc), felodipine (Plendil), isradipine (Dynacirc CR), nifedipine long-acting (Adalat CC, Procardia XL), nisoldipine (Sular)
- Adverse effects relevant to CKD: Constipation, nausea, edema

Alpha$_1$-Blockers
- Examples: doxazosin (Cardura), prazosin (Minipress), terazosin (Hytrin)
- Adverse effect relevant to CKD: Edema

Central Alpha$_2$-Agonists and Other Centrally Acting Drugs
- Examples: clonidine (Catapres), clonidin patch (Catapres-TTS), methyldopa (Aldomet), reserpine, guanfacine
- Adverse effects relevant to CKD: Dry mouth, nausea and vomiting, constipation, weight gain

Direct Vasodilators
- Examples: hydralazine (Apresoline), minoxidil (Loniten)
- Adverse effect relevant to CKD: Edema

Source: Data are from references 23 and 24.

Box 2.2   Phosphate-Binding Medications

Aluminum Hydroxide
- Forms: Liquid, tablet, capsule
- Mineral content: 100–200 mg aluminum per tablet
- Estimated potential binding capacity: 22.3 mg PO_4 bound per 5 mL; 14.3 mg PO_4 bound per tablet
- Potential advantages: Effective phosphate binder
- Potential disadvantages: Aluminum toxicity; altered bone mineral integrity; dementia. Not recommended except for very brief period secondary to danger of aluminum accumulation

Calcium Acetate
- Forms: Capsule, tablet
- Mineral content: 25% elemental calcium (250 mg Ca/g)
- Estimated potential binding capacity: 45 mg PO_4 bound per gram
- Potential advantages: Effective binder; less calcium load than $CaCO_3$ with same binding capacity
- Potential disadvantages: Increased potential for hypercalcemia and parathyroid (PTH) suppression; GI symptoms; large pill size

Calcium Carbonate
- Forms: Liquid, tablet, chewable, capsule, gum
- Mineral content: 40% elemental calcium (400 mg Ca/g)
- Estimated potential binding capacity: 39 mg of PO_4 bound per gram
- Potential advantages: Effective, inexpensive, and can be used as a calcium supplement
- Potential disadvantages: Increased calcium load with potential for hypercalcemia and PTH suppression; gastrointestinal (GI) symptoms

Calcium Citrate
- Form: Capsule, tablet
- Mineral content: 22% elemental calcium
- Estimated potential binding capacity: N/A
- Potential disadvantages: Not recommended; citrate enhances aluminum absorption and causes GI symptoms

(continued)

Box 2.2   Phosphate-Binding Medications (continued)

Lanthanum Carbonate
- Forms: Tablet, chewable
- Mineral content: 250 or 500 mg elemental lanthanum
- Estimated potential binding capacity: N/A
- Potential advantages: Effective
- Potential disadvantages: GI symptoms; cost; potential lanthanum accumulation

---

Magnesium Carbonate
- Forms: Capsule, tablet, liquid
- Mineral content: 28% magnesium
- Estimated potential binding capacity: N/A
- Potential advantages: Effective; potential for lower calcium load
- Potential disadvantages: GI symptoms; cost; potential for hypermagnesemia

---

Sevelamer Carbonate
- Forms: Tablet, powder
- Mineral content: None (does not contain calcium)
- Estimated potential binding capacity: N/A
- Potential advantages: Effective; not absorbed; potential to improve bicarbonate levels and decrease LDL cholesterol levels
- Potential disadvantages: GI symptoms; cost; large pill size

---

Sevelamer HCl
- Form: Tablet
- Mineral content: None (does not contain calcium)
- Estimated potential binding capacity: N/A
- Potential advantages: Effective; potential to lower LDL cholesterol levels; smaller tablet available for those with difficulty swallowing
- Potential disadvantages: GI symptoms; potential for decreased bicarbonate levels; cost; large size of 800-mg tab

---

N/A indicates that published data are not available.
Source: Data are from references 10 and 24.

Box 2.3   Hypoglycemic Agents and Recommendations for Use in Chronic Kidney Disease (CKD)

Insulin
- Dosing for CKD stage 3 or 4 or stage 5 nondialysis/kidney transplant: There is an increased risk of hypoglycemia due to decreased clearance of insulin by the kidney; adjust dose based on patient's/client's response.
- Dosing for dialysis: Adjust dose based on patient's/client's response.

First-Generation Sulfonylureas

Acetohexamide, tolazamide, and tolbutamide:
- Dosing for CKD stage 3 or 4 or stage 5 nondialysis/kidney transplant: Avoid.
- Dosing for dialysis: Avoid.

Chlorpropamide:
- Dosing for CKD stage 3 or 4 or stage 5 nondialysis/kidney transplant: Reduce dose by 50% when GFR is between <70 and ≥50 mL/min/1.73m^2; avoid when GFR is <50 mL/min/1.73 m^2.
- Dosing for dialysis: Avoid.

Second-Generation Sulfonylureas

Glipizide and gliclazide:
- Dosing for CKD stage 3 or 4 or stage 5 nondialysis/kidney transplant: No dose adjustment needed.
- Dosing for dialysis: No dose adjustment needed.

Glyburide and glimepiride:
- Dosing for CKD stage 3 or 4 or stage 5 nondialysis/kidney transplant: Avoid.
- Dosing for dialysis: Avoid.

Alpha-Glucosidase Inhibitors: Acarbose and Miglitol
- Dosing for CKD stage 3 or 4 or stage 5 nondialysis/kidney transplant: Not recommended if creatinine (Cr) >2 mg/dL.
- Dosing for dialysis: Avoid.

(continued)

**Box 2.3   Hypoglycemic Agents and Recommendations for Use
in Chronic Kidney Disease (CKD)** (continued)

Biguanides: Metformin
- Dosing for CKD stage 3 or 4 or stage 5 nondialysis/kidney transplant: Contraindicated with Cr ≥1.5 mg/dL in women or Cr ≥1.4 mg/dL in men.
- Dosing for dialysis: Avoid.

Meglitinides

Repaglinide:
- Dosing for CKD stage 3 or 4 or stage 5 nondialysis/kidney transplant: No dose adjustment needed.
- Dosing for dialysis: No dose adjustment needed.

Nateglinide:
- Dosing for CKD stage 3 or 4 or stage 5 nondialysis/kidney transplant: Initiate at low dose before meals.
- Dosing for dialysis: Avoid.

Thiazolidinediones: Pioglitazone and Rosiglitazone
- Dosing for CKD stage 3 or 4 or stage 5 nondialysis/kidney transplant: No dose adjustment needed.
- Dosing for dialysis: No dose adjustment needed.

Incretin Mimetic: Exenatide
- Dosing for CKD stage 3 or 4 or stage 5 nondialysis/kidney transplant: No dose adjustment needed.
- Dosing for dialysis: No dose adjustment needed.

Amylin Analog: Pramlintide
- Dosing for CKD stage 3 or 4 or stage 5 nondialysis/kidney transplant: No dose adjustment needed for GFR 20–50 mL/min/1.73m^2.
- Dosing for dialysis: No data available.

DPP-4 inhibitor: Sitagliptin
- Dosing for CKD stage 3 or 4 or stage 5 nondialysis/kidney transplant: Reduce dose by 50% with GFR <50 mL/min/1.73m^2, and by 75% when GFR is <30 mL/min/1.73m^2.
- Dosing for dialysis: Reduce dose by 75%.

Source: Data are from references 4 and 5.

Box 2.4 Dosing Adjustments for Medicines Used to Treat Lipid Disorders in Patients/Clients with Chronic Kidney Disease

Bile Acid Sequestrants
- Cholestyramine, colestipol, and colesevelam: No dose adjustment needed.

Statins
- Atorvastatin: No dose adjustment needed.
- Fluvastatin and lovastatin: Use caution with late-stage CKD. If GFR is <30 mL/min/1.73m^2, use caution with dose >20 mg/d.
- Pravastatin: No dose adjustment needed.
- Rosuvastatin: No dose adjustment needed with mild to moderate kidney disease. If GFR is <30 mL/min/1.73m^2, do not exceed 10 mg/d.
- Simvastatin: Initiate therapy at 5 mg/d in patients/clients with severe kidney disease.

Fibric Acid Derivatives
- Gemfibrozil: Decrease dose or consider alternative therapy if Cr is >2 mg/dL.
- Fenofibrate: Minimize dose in patients/clients with GFR <50 mL/min/1.73m^2.

Other
- Niacin and ezetimibe: No dose adjustments needed.

Source: Adapted from reference 4: National Kidney Foundation. KDOQI clinical practice guidelines and clinical practice recommendations for diabetes and chronic kidney disease. *Am J Kidney Dis.* 2007;49(2 suppl 2):S1–S180. www.kidney.org/professionals/KDOQI/guideline_diabetes. Adapted with permission from National Kidney Foundation, Inc.

Box 2.5   Possible Effects of Selected Drugs on Nutrient Absorption/Utilization

- Alcohol: Increased excretion of magnesium, potassium, and zinc; impaired utilization of folic acid.
- Antacids: Decreased absorption of phosphorus and iron; bicarbonate decreases folate and iron absorption.
- Antibiotics:
  - Cycloserine: Decreased levels of vitamins B-12, vitamin B-6, and folate.
  - Neomycin: Decreased absorption of fat; lactose; protein; vitamins A, D, K, and B-12; calcium; potassium; and iron.
  - Isoniazid: Pyridoxine (vitamin B-6) deficiency.
  - Tetracycline: Binds with calcium, magnesium, iron, and zinc.
  - Tobramycin: Increased urinary loss of potassium, magnesium.
- Anticoagulants: Decreased vitamin K–dependent coagulation factors.
- Anticonvulsants: Increased needs for vitamins K, D, and B-12; folic acid; calcium; and magnesium. Pyridoxine may increase drug effect.
- Anti-gout: Increased excretion of potassium, sodium, calcium, magnesium, amino acids, chloride, riboflavin (vitamin B-2).
- Anti-proliferative (azathioprine; mycophenolate): Nausea, vomiting, mucositis, altered taste. Folate deficiency; increased nutrient needs with infection. Possible bone marrow suppression in combination with anti-gout medications.
- Calcineurin inhibitors:
  - Cyclosporine A: Increases in serum potassium and glucose; hyperglycemia; hyperlipidemia.
  - Tacrolimus: Increased potassium and sodium retention; increased loss of magnesium; hyperglycemia.
- Corticosteroids: Hyperglycemia; increased protein catabolism or decreased protein synthesis; decreased absorption of calcium, phosphorus, and potassium; increased needs for vitamin B-6, folate, vitamins C and D, and zinc; impaired wound healing.
- Diuretics: Increased urinary excretion of magnesium, zinc, potassium, thiamin (B-1). **Note**: Spironolactone (acts in distal renal tubule) is potassium-sparing.

(continued)

Box 2.5   Possible Effects of Selected Drugs on Nutrient Absorption/Utilization (continued)

- Hypocholesterolemics: Decreased absorption of fat; carotene; vitamins A, D, K, and B-12; and iron.
- Laxatives: Increased fecal loss of fat, calcium, potassium, magnesium, fluids, most vitamins, carotene.
- Mineral oil: Decreased absorption of vitamins A, D, and E; potassium; and calcium. Effects may not be clinically significant.

Source: Data are from references 24 and 25.

ANTHROPOMETRIC MEASUREMENTS

The following weight standards may be used for CKD patients/clients (24):

- **Standard body weight (SBW)**: The median body weight for patients/clients of the same height, gender, frame size, and age from the National Health and Nutrition Examination Survey II (NHANES II) data (see Tables 2.3 to 2.6, in the Comparative Standards section later in this chapter).
- **Desirable body weight**: A weight determined using 1983 Metropolitan Life Insurance Height and Weight Tables.
- **Edema-free body weight (efBW)** or **dry weight**. To estimate dry weight:

$$\frac{142 \text{ mEq/L} \times \text{Liters of Normal Total Body Water}}{\text{Predialysis Serum Sodium (mEq/L)}}$$

$$= \text{Liters of Actual Body Water}$$

Where: Normal Total Body Water equals the predialysis weight multiplied by the average percentage of body water for males (60%) or for females (50%).

If the patient/client has muscle-wasting or is overweight, multiply the predialysis weight by 57% for males or 47% for females.

- **Adjusted body weight (ABW)**: ABW is used for a lean or obese patient/client whose weight is less than 95% or greater than 115% standard body weight (3). See Box 2.9, later in this chapter, for information on how to calculate ABW.

The Academy's systematic review of the literature on anthropometric assessment in patients/clients with CKD stages 1 through 5 (nondialysis) identified the following recommendations (2):

- Use clinical judgment in assessing body weight. There is a lack of standard reference norms for this population; therefore, clinical judgment must be used when determining which weight to use in assessment—ie, actual measured weight, history of weight changes, serial weight measurements, or weight adjusted for edema.
- Use published weight norms with caution. Ideal body weight, the Hamwi method to determine optimal body weight, standard body weight, body mass index (BMI), and adjusted body weight all have drawbacks in the assessment of body weight in patients/clients with CKD.
- In the assessment of body composition, consider that CKD patients/clients have altered body composition compared to healthy individuals.
- In body composition assessment, use valid measurements methodology, such as anthropometrics (including waist circumference and BMI) and body compartment estimates; there are no reference

standards for assessing body composition in this population.

Obesity is a common problem in patients/clients with CKD, as it is with the population as a whole. Table 2.1 lists the BMI classification system for obesity (26), and Box 2.6 lists the proposed mechanisms for the association between obesity and CKD (4).

Table 2.1 International Classification of Adult Weight According to Body Mass Index (BMI)

	BMI	
Classification	Principal Cut-off Points	Additional Cut-off Points[a]
Underweight	<18.50	<18.50
Severe thinness	<16.00	<16.00
Moderate thinness	16.00–16.99	16.00–16.99
Mild thinness	17.00–18.49	17.00–18.49
Normal range	18.50–24.99	18.50–22.99
		23.00–24.99
Overweight	≥25.00	≥25.00
Pre-obese	25.00–29.99	25.00–27.49
		27.50–29.99
Obese	≥30.00	≥30.00
Obese class I	30.00–34.99	30.00–32.49
		32.50–34.99
Obese class II	35.00–39.99	35.00–37.49
		37.50–39.99
Obese class III	≥40.00	≥40.00

[a]Points for public health action.
Source: Data are from reference 26.

Box 2.6   Proposed Mechanisms for the Association between Obesity and Chronic Kidney Disease (CKD)

- Physical compression of the kidneys
- Renal angiotension system activation
- Hyperinsulinemia
- Sympathetic activation
- Overnutrition
- Glomerular hyperfiltration
- Proteinuria-associated kidney damage
- Blood pressure elevation

Source: Adapted from reference 4: National Kidney Foundation. KDOQI clinical practice guidelines and clinical practice recommendations for diabetes and chronic kidney disease. *Am J Kidney Dis.* 2007;49(suppl 2):S1–S180. Adapted with permission from National Kidney Foundation, Inc.

BIOCHEMICAL DATA, MEDICAL TESTS, AND DIAGNOSTIC CRITERIA

To accurately assess the ramifications of the various biochemical data that are affected by CKD, the registered dietitian (RD) must understand the stages of CKD (see Table 1.1 in Chapter 1) and their effect on nutrition assessment. These biochemical data are directly related to the metabolic abnormalities of CKD: anemia, bone and mineral abnormalities, electrolyte imbalances, hyperglycemia, inflammation, protein-energy malnutrition, acid-base balance, and fluid balance. Box 2.7 relates biochemical parameters to the metabolic conditions of CKD (2). Accepted values for each of these parameters as well as the frequency of measurements for some may change with the stage of CKD, as described in Box 2.8 (24) and Table 2.2 (10).

Box 2.7   Biochemical Data Used in Nutrition Assessment of Patients/Clients with Chronic Kidney Disease (CKD)

Anemia Assessment
- Hemoglobin (Hgb)
- Serum transferrin saturation (TSAT) or reticulocyte hemoglobin content (CHr)
- Mean corpuscular hemoglobin (MCH)
- Mean corpuscular volume (MCV)[a]
- Differential and platelet count [a]
- Serum iron (Fe)
- Serum ferritin
- Total iron-binding capacity (TIBC)
- Absolute reticulocyte count
- Red blood cell (RBC) folate
- Serum vitamin B-12
- White blood cell count[a]

Bone Health Assessment
- Serum phosphorus (PO_4)
- Serum calcium (Ca), corrected
- Serum calcium–phosphorus product ($Ca \times PO_4$)
- Intact plasma parathyroid hormone (iPTH)
- Serum 25-hydroxyvitamin D

Dyslipidemia Assessment
- Total cholesterol
- Low-density lipoprotein (LDL)
- High-density lipoprotein (HDL)
- Triglycerides

Electrolyte Balance Assessment
- Serum albumin (Alb)
- Serum sodium (Na)
- Serum potassium (K)
- Serum carbon dioxide (CO_2)
- Home capillary blood glucose (CBG) records[a]

(continued)

**Box 2.7   Biochemical Data Used in Nutrition Assessment of
           Patients/Clients with Chronic Kidney Disease (CKD)**
           (continued)

Glycemia Assessment
- Home CBGs
- Hgb A1c
- Serum glucose (random, fasting, preprandial, postprandial)
- Triglycerides[a]

Inflammation Assessment
- Serum Alb
- C-reactive protein (CRP)
- White blood cell count (WBC)
- Serum ferritin
- Serum Fe[a]
- TIBC[a]
- Absolute reticulocyte count[a]

Kidney Function Assessment
- Estimated glomerular filtration rate (eGFR)
- Creatinine clearance rate, 24-hour
- Proteinuria
- Proteinuria, g/24 hours
- Urinary microalbumin-to-creatinine ratio (MAC)
- Glomerular filtration (Glofil)
- Serum creatinine (Cr)
- Blood urea nitrogen (BUN)
- Serum PO_4
- Serum magnesium (Mg)
- Home CBGs[a]

Protein Energy Malnutrition Assessment
- Proteinuria
- Proteinuria, g/24 hours
- Urinary MAC
- Serum Cr
- Normalized protein nitrogen appearance (nPNA)
- Serum albumin
- Serum prealbumin (serum transthyretin)

(continued)

Box 2.7 Biochemical Data Used in Nutrition Assessment of Patients/Clients with Chronic Kidney Disease (CKD) (continued)

Protein Energy Malnutrition Assessment (continued)
- Home CBGs[a]
- Total cholesterol[a]
- TIBC [a]

Assessment of Other Conditions[a]
- Serum Alb
- Serum Na
- Serum 25-hydroxyvitamin D
- Serum Mg[a]

---

[a]Secondary marker, additional interpretations may be appropriate.
Source: Data are from reference 2.

Box 2.8 Interpretation of Biochemical Data in Patients/Clients with Chronic Kidney Disease (CKD)

Albumin
- Reference range: 3.5–5.0 g/dL
- CKD range: Within normal limits (WNL) for the laboratory
- Interpretation of abnormal values:
  - High: May indicate severe dehydration.
  - Low: May indicate fluid overload, infection, chronic liver disease, steatorrhea, nephrotic syndrome, protein-energy malnutrition, or inflammatory GI disease.

Alkaline Phosphatase
- Reference range: 30–85 IU/L
- CKD range: WNL
- Interpretation of abnormal values:
  - High: May indicate renal osteodystrophy, malignancy, healing fractures, or liver disease.
  - Low: May indicate congenital hypophosphatemia or nephrotic syndrome.

(continued)

**Box 2.8   Interpretation of Biochemical Data in Patients/Clients
with Chronic Kidney Disease (CKD)** (continued)

Aluminum
- Reference range: <7 mcg/L
- CKD range: <20 mcg/L
- Interpretation of abnormal values:
  - High: May indicate ingestion of aluminum-containing medications. Other possible sources of aluminum include parenteral fluids, injections, antiperspirants, or dialysates.
  - If >60 mcg/L, perform deferoxamine (DFO) test.

B-12
- Reference range: 100–700 pg/mL
- CKD range: WNL
- Interpretation of abnormal values:
  - High: May indicate leukemia, polycythemia vera, or severe liver dysfunction.
  - Low: May indicate pernicious anemia, atrophic gastritis, malabsorption syndrome, inflammatory bowel disease, or vitamin C or folic acid deficiency.

Blood Urea Nitrogen (BUN)
- Reference range: 10–20 mg/dL
- CKD range: 60–80 mg/dL
- Interpretation of abnormal values:
  - High: May indicate GI bleeding, dehydration, hyper-catabolism, congestive heart failure, transplant rejection, inadequate dialysis, or excessive protein intake.
  - Low: May indicate liver failure, over hydration, mal-absorption, acute protein intake, elevated secretion of anabolic hormones, or residual renal function.

Creatinine
- Reference range: Women: 0.5–1.1 mg/dL; men: 0.6–1.2 mg/dL
- CKD range: 2–15 mg/dL (based on muscle mass, GFR, and/or dialysis clearance)
- Interpretation of abnormal values:
  - High: May indicate muscle damage, catabolism, myocardial infarction, acute kidney injury, chronic kidney disease, inadequate dialysis, or transplant rejection.

(continued)

Box 2.8 Interpretation of Biochemical Data in Patients/Clients with Chronic Kidney Disease (CKD) (continued)

Creatinine (continued)
- ○ Low: <10 mg/dL in chronic dialysis may indicate protein-energy malnutrition/muscle wasting or residual renal function.

Ferritin
- Reference range: Men: 12–300 ng/mL;
  women: 10–150 ng/mL
- CKD range: Hemodialysis ≥20 ng/mL; peritoneal dialysis >100 ng/mL
- Interpretation of abnormal values:
  - ○ High: May indicate iron overload, transfusions, dehydration, or inflammatory state; values may be falsely elevated in active liver disease.
  - ○ Low: May indicate iron deficiency.

Folic Acid
- Reference range: 5–20 mcg/mL
- CKD range: WNL
- Interpretation of abnormal values:
  - ○ High: May indicate pernicious anemia or recent blood transfusions.
  - ○ Low: May indicate folic acid deficiency, hemolytic anemia, malnutrition, malabsorption, malignancy, liver disease, pregnancy, alcoholism, or anorexia nervosa.

Glucose (Fasting)
- Reference range: 70–105 mg/dL
- CKD range: WNL
- Interpretation of abnormal values:
  - ○ High: May indicate diabetes, chronic hepatic disease, hyperthyroidism, malignancy, acute stress, burns, or pancreatic insufficiency.
  - ○ Low: May indicate hyperinsulinemia, alcohol abuse, pancreatic tumors, liver failure, pituitary dysfunction, malnutrition, or extreme exercise.

(continued)

Box 2.8 Interpretation of Biochemical Data in Patients/Clients with Chronic Kidney Disease (CKD) (continued)

Hematocrit
- Reference range: Men: 42%–52%; women: 37%–47%
- CKD range: Men: 33%–36%; women: <39%
- Interpretation of abnormal values:
  - High: May indicate polycythemia or dehydration.
  - Low: May indicate anemias, blood loss, CKD, or insufficient erythropoiesis-stimulating agent (ESA).

Iron
- Reference range: Men: 60–175 mcg/dL; women: 50–170 mcg/dL
- CKD range: WNL
- Interpretation of abnormal values:
  - High: May indicate iron overload or hemolysis.
  - Low: May indicate iron deficiency, decreased iron intake, or blood loss.

Lipoproteins
- Reference range:
  - HDL: Men: >45 mg/dL; women: >55 mg/dL
  - LDL: 60–180 mg/dL
  - VLDL: 25–50 mg/dL
- CKD range: WNL
- Interpretation of abnormal values:
  - High HDL: May indicate familial lipoproteinemia or excessive exercise.
  - High LDL/VLDL: May indicate familial lipoproteinemia, nephrotic syndrome, hypothyroidism, chronic liver disease, or poor glycemic control.
  - Low HDL: May indicate familial hypolipoproteinemia, hepatocellular disease, or hypoproteinemia.
  - Low LDL/VLDL: May indicate familial hypolipoproteinemia or hypoproteinemia due to severe burns, malabsorption, or malnutrition.

Magnesium
- Reference range: 1.2–2.0 mEq/L
- CKD range: WNL

(continued)

Box 2.8   Interpretation of Biochemical Data in Patients/Clients with Chronic Kidney Disease (CKD) (continued)

Magnesium (continued)
- Interpretation of abnormal values:
  - High: May indicate excessive magnesium intake from water, dialysate, magnesium-containing medications, or parenteral infusion; may also indicate dehydration.
  - Low: May indicate ketoacidosis, hypercalcemia, some diuretics, alcohol abuse, refeeding syndrome, diarrhea/malabsorption, or malnutrition.

Mean Corpuscular Volume (MCV)
- Reference range: 80–95μm³
- CKD range: WNL
- Interpretation of abnormal values:
  - High: May indicate folic acid or vitamin B-12 deficiency, cirrhosis, reticulocytosis, chronic alcoholism, or adverse effects of medications (eg, some chemotherapy agents and some immunosuppressants).
  - Low: May indicate chronic iron deficiency or anemia of chronic disease.

Prealbumin
- Reference range: 15–36 mg/dL
- CKD range: ≥30 mg/dL
- Interpretation of abnormal values:
  - High: May indicate use of corticosteroids.
  - Low: May indicate liver disease, malnutrition, or inflammation.

Intact Parathyroid Hormone (iPTH)
- Reference range: 10–65 pg/mL
- CKD range: KDOQI: 150–300 pg/mL; KDIGO: 2–9 times normal limit
- Interpretation of abnormal values:
  - High: May indicate hyperparathyroidism, non-PTH producing tumors, lung or kidney cancer, hypocalcemia, malabsorption, vitamin D deficiency, rickets.
  - Low: May indicate hypoparathyroidism, hypercalcemia, metastatic bone tumor, sarcoidosis, vitamin D intoxication, hypomagnesemia.

Source: Data are from reference 24.

**Table 2.2   Frequency of Measures to Evaluate Metabolic
Bone Disease (MBD) in Patients/Clients with
Chronic Kidney Disease (CKD)**

	Progressive CKD Stage 3	CKD Stage 4	CKD Stages 5 and 5D
Calcium and phosphorus	6–12 months	3–6 months	1–3 months
PTH and alkaline phosphatases	Baseline	6–12 months	3–6 months
Calcidiol (25 hydroxy-vitamin D)	Baseline	Baseline	Baseline

Source: Reprinted from reference 10: Kidney Disease: Improving Global Outcomes (KDIGO) CKD-MBD Work Group. KDIGO clinical practice guidelines for the diagnosis, evaluation, prevention, and treatment of chronic kidney disease-mineral and bone disorder (CKD-MBD). *Kidney Int.* 2009; 76 (suppl 113):S1–S130. www.kdigo.org/clinical_practice_guidelines/kdigo_guideline _for_ckd-mbd.php. Reprinted with permission from National Kidney Foundation, Inc.

NUTRITION-FOCUSED PHYSICAL FINDINGS

The fourth edition of the *IDNT Reference Manual* outlines numerous factors to consider when gathering and interpreting nutrition-focused physical findings as part of a complete nutrition assessment (1). Examples of potential findings in CKD include:

- Overall appearance: eg, cushingoid appearance; amputations, specify; affect, specify
- Body language (note: varies by culture), specify (eg, body positioning; eye contact)
- Cardiovascular-pulmonary system: eg, edema; shortness of breath; interdialytic weight gain
- Extremities, muscles and bones: eg, edema, peripheral (specify); fat, subcutaneous, specify excess or

loss; feeling cold all of the time; muscle mass, specify; nails, nail beds, specify: blue, clubbing, pale, other; weakness; cramping

- Digestive system: eg, excessive belching; cheilosis; xerostomia; gingivitis; heartburn; ketone smell on breath; oral lesions; dry or cracked lips; altered mastication; polydipsia; stomatitis; compromised or painful swallow function; taste alteration, specify; teeth, specify (edentulous, partially or completely); tongue, specify: bright red, magenta, dry cracked, glossitis, impaired movement, frenulum abnormality; appetite, specify; ascites; bowel function, including flatus, specify (eg, type, frequency, volume); epigastric pain; nausea; satiety, specify; vomiting
- Head and eyes: bitot's spots; night blindness; jaundiced sclera; xerophthalmia; hair, specify: brittle, lifeless, coiled, loss; altered olfactory sense, specify; temporal wasting
- Nerves and cognition: eg, gait disturbance; confusion
- Skin: calcinosis; dry; follicular hyperkeratosis; poor turgor; petechiae; pressure ulcers; poor wound healing; xanthomas
- Vital signs: eg, blood pressure; heart rate; temperature

CLIENT HISTORY

Client data to be gathered and considered in the nutrition assessment include social history; personal medical and health history, including comorbid conditions; demographic information; and family medical history, with a focus on conditions that might lead to a higher risk of kidney disease, including diabetes, hypertension, hyperlipidemia, and kidney stones. Assessment of the patient's/client's current level of physical activity and any known reasons that physical activity is contraindicated will also assist in developing the nutrition prescription.

COMPARATIVE STANDARDS

This section presents established guidelines for standard body weight for men and women (Tables 2.3 to 2.6) (27), adjusted body weight for obese and underweight CKD patients/clients (Box 2.9) (24), amputation adjustments (Table 2.7) (28), and energy needs during acute illness (Table 2.8) (24).

Table 2.3   NHANES II Standard Body Weight (SBW) for Men Ages 25–54 Years

Height, cm	SBW for Frame Size, kg		
	Small	Medium	Large
157	64	68	82
160	61	71	83
163	66	71	84
165	66	74	79
168	67	75	84
170	71	77	84
173	71	78	86
175	74	78	89
178	75	81	87
180	76	81	91
183	74	84	91
185	79	85	93
188	80	88	92

Source: Data are from reference 27.

Table 2.4　NHANES II Standard Body Weight (SBW) for Men Ages 55–74 Years

Height, cm	SBW for Frame Size, kg		
	Small	Medium	Large
157	61	68	77
160	62	70	80
163	63	71	77
165	70	72	79
168	68	74	80
170	69	72	85
173	70	72	86
175	75	77	84
178	76	80	87
180	69	84	84
183	76	81	90
185	78	88	88
188	77	95	89

Source: Data are from reference 27.

Table 2.5　NHANES II Standard Body Weight (SBW) for Women Ages 25–54 Years

Height, cm	SBW for Frame Size, kg		
	Small	Medium	Large
147	52	63	86
150	53	66	78
152	53	60	87
155	54	61	81
157	55	61	81
160	55	62	8
163	57	62	79

(continued)

**Table 2.5   NHANES II Standard Body Weight
(SBW) for Women Ages 25–54 Years** (continued)

Height, cm	SBW for Frame Size, kg		
	Small	Medium	Large
165	60	63	81
168	58	63	75
170	59	65	80
173	62	67	76
175	62	68	79
178	64	70	76

Source: Data are from reference 27.

**Table 2.6   NHANES II Standard Body Weight
(SBW) for Women Ages 55–74 Years**

Height, cm	SBW for Frame Size, kg		
	Small	Medium	Large
147	54	57	92
150	55	62	78
152	54	65	78
155	56	64	79
157	58	64	82
160	58	65	80
163	60	66	77
165	60	67	80
168	68	66	82
170	61	72	80
173	61	70	79
175	62	72	85
178	63	73	85

Source: Data are from reference 27.

Box 2.9   Adjusted Body Weight (ABW) for Obese and Underweight Chronic Kidney Disease (CKD) Patients/Clients

ABW should be used when a patient's/client's weight is <95% or >115% of standard body weight (SBW). (See Tables 2.3–2.6 for SBWs.) There is no conclusive scientific evidence regarding which formula for ABW (KDOQI vs traditional) should be used in patients/clients with CKD.

KDOQI Formula

$$ABW = \text{Edema-free body weight (BW)}$$
$$+ [(SBW - \text{Edema-free BW}) \times 0.25]$$

Where: Body weight is measured in kilograms.
Example: CKD patient/client whose edema-free body weight is 72 kg.

$$ABW = 72 \text{ kg} + [(62 \text{ kg} - 72 \text{ kg}) \times 0.25]$$
$$= 72 \text{ kg} - 2.5 \text{ kg}$$
$$= 69.5 \text{ kg}$$

Traditional Formula

$$ABW = \text{Ideal body weight (IBW)}$$
$$+ [(\text{Actual BW} - IBW) \times 0.25]$$

Where: Body weight is measured in kilograms and IBW is defined as:
- Men: 48.1 kg for first 152.4 cm, plus 1.1 kg for every centimeter above 152.4 cm (106 lb for the first 5 feet plus 6 lb for each inch over 5 feet)
- Women: 45.5 kg for first 152.4 cm, plus 0.9 kg for every centimeter above 152.4 cm (100 pounds for the first 5 feet plus 5 pounds for each inch over 5 feet)

Example: CKD patient/client whose actual body weight is 72 kg and IBW is 43.2 kg.

$$ABW = 43.2 \text{ kg} + [(72 \text{ kg} - 43.2 \text{ kg}) \times 0.25]$$
$$= 43.2 \text{ kg} + 7.2 \text{ kg}$$
$$= 50.4 \text{ kg}$$

Source: Data are from reference 24.

Table 2.7 Amputation Adjustments

Body Segment	Average Percentage (%) of Total Body Weight
Entire arm	5.0
Upper arm (to elbow)	2.7
Forearm	1.3
Hand	0.7
Entire leg	16.0
Thigh	10.1
Calf	4.4
Foot	1.5

Source: Reprinted with permission from reference 28: Wiggins KL. *Guidelines for Nutrition Care of Renal Patients.* Chicago, IL: American Dietetic Association; 2001.

Table 2.8 Suggested Adjustment Factors for Energy Needs During Acute Illness

Condition	Adjustment Factor
Bone fracture	1.2–1.25
Burns (% burned)	
0%–20%	1.0–1.5
21%–40%	1.5–1.95
41%–100%	1.85–2.05
Elective surgery	
Day 1–4	1.0
Day 18–21	0.95
Fever	0.07 (7%) per °F above normal
	0.13 (13%) per °C above normal

(continued)

Table 2.8   Suggested Adjustment Factors for Energy Needs During Acute Illness (continued)

Condition	Adjustment Factor
Infection	
Mild	1.0
Moderate	1.2–1.4
Severe	1.4–1.6
Maintenance hemodialysis	1.0–1.05
Multiple organ failure	1.2–1.4
Nondialyzed CKD	1.0
Peritonitis, soft tissue trauma	1.15
Postoperative (no complications)	1.0
Postoperative (with complications)	1.2–1.25

Source: Data are from reference 24.

CASE STUDY—NCP STEP 1: ASSESSMENT

This case involves a 56-year-old Cambodian woman with ESRD. The nutrition assessment is presented here. Later chapters continue to develop the case with information appropriate to each step of the NCP.

Food/Nutrition-Related History

- FH 1.2.2 Food intake: Traditional Cambodian foods and meal patterns: rice and stir-fried vegetables, small amounts fish, poultry, beef. Uses fish sauce.
- FH 3.1 Medications: Atorvastatin; renal multivitamin; calcium carbonate and Renagel with meals; calcitriol; ferrous sulfate; NPH insulin with meals; isoniazid; vitamin B-6; lansoprazole.

- FH 4.1 Food and nutrition knowledge/skill: Family is aware of low-phosphorus and low-potassium foods; very involved.
- FH 7.3 Physical activity: Sedentary.

Anthropometric Measurements

- AD 1.1 Body composition/growth/weight history:
  ◦ Height: 59 inches (150 cm)
  ◦ Admitting weight: 74.5 kg
  ◦ Estimated dry weight (EDW): 72 kg (has been stable)
  ◦ BMI (using EDW): 32
  ◦ Frame size: medium (SBW 62 kg; patient is 116% SBW)

Biochemical Data, Medical Tests, and Procedures

- BD 1.2 Electrolyte and renal profile: see Table 2.9 (24)
- BD 1.10 Nutritional anemia profile: see Table 2.9 (24)
- BD 1.12.5 Urine volume: 500 mL/24 hours

Table 2.9   Laboratory Data for Nutrition Assessment of Case Study Patient

Laboratory Test	Reference Ranges[a]	Patient's Result
K, mmol/L	Normal: 3.4–5.0 PD: 3.5–5.5	5.4
BUN, mg/dL	Normal: 6–20 PD: >60	58
Cr, mg/dL	Normal: 0.7–1.3 PD: Not defined	11.0
Glucose, mg/dL	Normal: 60–99	92
Ca, mg/dL	Normal: 8.6–10.2	8.8

(continued)

Table 2.9 Laboratory Data for Nutrition Assessment of Case Study Patient (continued)

Laboratory Test	Reference Ranges[a]	Patient's Result
PO_4, mg/dL	Normal: 2.4–4.7 PD: 3.5–5.5	5.7
Alb, g/dL	Normal: 3.5–4.7 PD: >3.5	1.6
Hgb, g/dL	Normal: 13.5–17.5 PD: 10–12	9.0
Capillary blood glucose, mg/dL	Normal: <150	120–250
Na, mmol/L	Normal: 134–143	129

[a]PD = Reference range for patients on peritoneal dialysis.
Source: Data are from reference 24.

Nutrition-Focused Physical Findings

- PD 1.1.1 Overall appearance: Obese; abrasions on arms, neck from scratching
- PD 1.1.4 Extremities, muscles, bones: Bilateral lower-extremity edema (LEE)
- PD 1.1.6 Head and eyes: Facial edema

Client History

- CH 1.1 Personal data: 56-year-old woman, Cambodian (speaks Cambodian; children fluent in English). Children very involved, supportive.
- CH 2.1 Patient/client medical/health history: ESRD due to hypertension (HTN). History includes type 2 diabetes mellitus. Admitted with peritonitis, pain, nausea and vomiting, fever. Third episode of peritonitis in 2 months. Latent tuberculosis.
- CH 2.2.1 Medical treatment/therapy: Peritoneal dialysis with 5 exchanges per day, each 2 liters of 2.5% dextrose. Type 2 diabetes mellitus managed with insulin; CBG usually <250 mg/dL.

Chapter 3

Nutrition Diagnosis

The nutrition diagnosis provides a formal label for the nutrition problem that has been identified from information gathered during the nutrition assessment. The diagnosis should follow the International Dietetics and Nutrition Terminology (IDNT) standardized terminology for nutrition diagnoses (1). As described in the Nutrition Care Process and Model (NCPM), the diagnosis is based on data collected in the nutrition assessment and evaluated by the registered dietitian (RD) in the context of clinical experience and practice guidelines. Following the nutrition diagnosis, the next steps of the Nutrition Care Process (NCP) are nutrition intervention (see Chapters 4 and 5); and monitoring and evaluation (see Chapter 6).

Medical diagnoses describe medical conditions that are treated by a licensed independent practitioner (eg, a physician or nurse practitioner). On the other hand, *nutrition* diagnoses describe problems of a nutritional origin, which are clearly related to an individual's nutritional status and which are treated by nutrition interventions directed by RDs.

The IDNT nutrition diagnosis terminology is organized into three categories (1):

- Intake: "Actual problems related to intake of energy, nutrients, fluids, and bioactive substances through

oral diet or nutrition support (enteral or parenteral nutrition)."
- Clinical: "Nutritional findings/problems that relate to medical or physical conditions."
- Behavioral-Environmental: "Nutritional findings/problems identified that relate to knowledge, attitudes/beliefs, physical environment, access to food, or food safety."

PROBLEM, ETIOLOGY, SIGNS AND SYMPTOMS STATEMENTS

After a nutrition diagnosis has been established, the RD develops a nutrition diagnostic statement, also called a "problem, etiology, signs and symptoms (PES) statement." This concise statement identifies the diagnosis (problem) and links it to an etiology and to signs and symptoms (1).

A well-written PES statement follows this format: Problem *related to* etiology, *as evidenced by* signs and symptoms (1).

- The *problem* is taken from the IDNT standardized nutrition diagnosis terminology. More than one problem may be diagnosed for a particular patient/client. Every problem that is identified must be addressed in the intervention and monitoring and evaluation steps of the NCP.
- The *etiology* describes the underlying cause of the diagnosis. For example, an etiology such as "lack of prior nutrition education" suggests that the intervention will include education or counseling about the problem, whereas an etiology such as "overfeeding of parenteral/enteral nutrition" might indicate the

need to adjust the nutrition support regimen. Thus, as stated earlier, the etiology leads to an intervention.

- The *signs and symptoms* in a PES statement are data elements from the assessment that support the diagnosis. Moving forward, the signs and symptoms are the parameters that will be followed to measure progress toward the goals that are established in the patient's/client's nutrition care plan.

The rest of this chapter presents general suggestions for nutrition diagnoses and PES statements that may apply in patients/clients with chronic kidney disease (CKD) or end-stage renal disease (ESRD). These are followed by suggested nutrition diagnoses for the case study introduced in Chapter 2.

SAMPLE PES STATEMENTS IN CKD

Boxes 3.1 to 3.3, which are arranged by IDNT domain, offer common examples of nutrition diagnoses for patients with CKD, along with corresponding PES statements (1).

Box 3.1   Selected Intake Domain Nutrition Diagnoses for Patients/Clients with Chronic Kidney Disease (CKD)

Excessive Energy Intake
- Definition: Energy intake that exceeds expenditure, established reference standards, or recommendations based on physiological needs.
- Sample PES statement: Excessive energy intake related to energy from peritoneal dialysate plus diet as evidenced by total intake exceeding estimated needs of 35 kcal/kg/d.

(continued)

Box 3.1 Selected Intake Domain Nutrition Diagnoses for Patients/Clients with Chronic Kidney Disease (CKD)
(continued)

Inadequate Energy Intake
- Definition: Energy intake that is less than energy expenditure, established reference standards, or recommendations based on physiological needs.
- Sample PES statement: Inadequate energy intake related to decreased appetite in patient with uremic symptoms as evidenced by average daily intake <50% of estimated needs.

Inadequate Oral Intake
- Definition: Oral food/beverage intake that is less than established reference standards or recommendations based on physiological needs.
- Sample PES statement: Inadequate oral intake related to poor appetite in patient with uremia, as evidenced by food recall showing about 50% of estimated energy needs.

Excessive Fluid Intake
- Definition: Higher intake of fluid compared to established reference standards or recommendations based on physiologic needs.
- Sample PES statement: Excessive fluid intake related to patient not adjusting for reduced urine output as evidenced by patient continuing 2–3 liters of fluid intake per day despite urine output <1 L/d.

Increased Nutrient Needs (Protein)
- Definition: Increased need for a specific nutrient compared to established reference standards or recommendations based on physiological needs.
- Sample PES statement: Increased protein needs related to increased demand for protein as evidenced by patient starting peritoneal dialysis.

(continued)

**Box 3.1   Selected Intake Domain Nutrition Diagnoses for
            Patients/Clients with Chronic Kidney Disease (CKD)**
            (continued)

Malnutrition
- Definition: Inadequate intake of protein and/or energy over
  prolonged periods of time resulting in loss of fat stores
  and/or muscle stores, including starvation-related malnutrition, chronic disease– or condition-related malnutrition, and
  acute disease– or injury-related malnutrition.
- Sample PES statement: Malnutrition related to food- and
  nutrition-related knowledge deficit as evidenced by unintentional weight loss (>7.5% in 3 months) and loss of orbital
  and triceps fat in patient on severe self-imposed diet with 30
  gram protein per day during CKD stage 4.

**Excessive Mineral Intake (Examples: Potassium,
Phosphorus)**
- Definition: Higher intake of a specified mineral(s) compared
  to established reference standards or recommendations
  based on physiologic needs.
- Sample PES statements:
  ○ Excessive potassium intake related to patient enjoy-
    ing seasonal produce as evidenced by elevated serum
    potassium and reported intake of fresh tomatoes.
  ○ Excessive phosphorus intake related to patient with nutri-
    tion-related knowledge deficit as evidenced by new diag-
    nosis of CKD and 24-hour food recall showing multiple
    high-phosphorus foods at each meal.

Excessive Vitamin Intake
- Definition: Higher intake of one or more vitamins compared
  to established reference standards or recommendations
  based on physiological needs.
- Sample PES statement: Excessive vitamin C intake related
  to food- and nutrition-related knowledge deficit as evidenced
  by individual with CKD stage 4 consuming 1,000 mg vitamin C per day.

Source: Data are from reference 1.

Box 3.2   Selected Clinical Domain Nutrition Diagnoses for Patients/Clients with Chronic Kidney Disease (CKD)

Impaired Nutrient Utilization
- Definition: Changes in ability to metabolize nutrients and bioactive substances.
- Sample PES statements:
  - Impaired potassium utilization related to reduced excretion at eGFR 10 mL/min/1.73 m^2, as evidenced by elevated serum potassium in patient adhering to low-potassium diet.
  - Impaired glucose utilization related to medication side effects as evidenced by capillary blood glucose levels >180 in posttransplant patient on tacrolimus.

Altered Nutrition-Related Laboratory Values (Specify)
- Definition: Changes due to body composition, medications, body system changes or genetics, or changes in ability to eliminate byproducts of digestive and metabolic processes.
- Sample PES statement: Altered nutrition-related laboratory value (serum phosphorus) related to changes in mineral elimination in ESRD, as evidenced by elevated serum phosphorus in CKD Stage 5 patient (pre-dialysis) who previously controlled serum phosphorus by diet.

Food-Medication Interaction
- Definition: Undesirable harmful interaction(s) between food and over-the-counter (OTC) medications, prescribed medications, herbals, botanicals, and/or dietary supplements that diminishes, enhances, or alters the effect of nutrients and/or medications.
- Sample PES statement: Food-medication interaction related to post–kidney transplant patient resuming St. John's wort while on tacrolimus for immunosuppression as evidenced by new onset of subtherapeutic tacrolimus levels.

Unintended Weight Loss
- Definition: Decrease in body weight that is not planned or desired.

(continued)

**Box 3.2   Selected Clinical Domain Nutrition Diagnoses for
             Patients/Clients with Chronic Kidney Disease (CKD)**
             (continued)

Unintended Weight Loss (continued)
- Sample PES statement: Unintentional weight loss related
  to food aversions as evidenced by patient describing many
  foods that she began to dislike in the last month while eGFR
  declined sharply.

Unintended Weight Gain
- Definition: Weight gain more than that which is desired or
  planned.
- Sample PES statement: Unintentional weight gain related to
  decreased activity and peritoneal dialysate energy absorption
  as evidenced by 7 kg (10%) weight gain since starting PD.

Source: Data are from reference 1.

**Box 3.3   Selected Behavioral-Environmental Domain Nutrition
             Diagnoses for Patients/Clients with Chronic Kidney
             Disease (CKD)**

Food- and Nutrition-Related Knowledge Deficit
- Definition: Incomplete or inaccurate knowledge about food,
  nutrition, or nutrition-related information and guidelines.
- Sample PES statement: Food- and nutrition-related knowledge deficit related to no prior education regarding diet for
  CKD as evidenced by client with many questions about diet
  and self-report of no nutrition education.

**Unsupported Beliefs/Attitudes about Food or
Nutrition-Related Topics**
- Definition: *Use with caution. Be sensitive to patient/cli-
  ent concerns.* Beliefs, attitudes, or practices about food,
  nutrition, and nutrition-related topics that are incompatible
  with sound nutrition principles, nutrition care, or disease/
  condition (excluding disordered eating patterns and eating
  disorders).

(continued)

Box 3.3   Selected Behavioral-Environmental Domain Nutrition Diagnoses for Patients/Clients with Chronic Kidney Disease (CKD) (continued)

Unsupported Beliefs/Attitudes about Food or Nutrition-Related Topics (continued)
- Sample PES statement: Unsupported beliefs/attitudes about food or nutrition-related topics related to patient with pica-like behavior as evidenced by reported intense cravings and subsequent intake of 1 large bag of ice cubes per day and interdialytic weight gains of 5 to 7 kg.

Self-Monitoring Deficit
- Definition: Lack of data recording to track personal progress.
- Sample PES statement: Self-monitoring deficit related to patient not ready for diet-lifestyle change as evidenced by no progress on suggested monitoring tool after education and encouragement from multiple dialysis team members.

Limited Adherence to Nutrition-Related Recommendations
- Definition: Lack of nutrition-related changes as per intervention agreed upon by client or population.
- Sample PES statement: Limited adherence to nutrition-related recommendations related to lack of support for implementing changes as evidenced by patient's inconsistent use of phosphorus binders and rising serum phosphorus.

Undesirable Food Choices
- Definition: Food and/or beverage choices inconsistent with dietary reference intake standards (eg, Dietary Reference Intakes), national food guidelines (eg, US Dietary Guidelines, MyPlate), diet quality index standards (eg, Healthy Food Index), or as defined in the nutrition prescription.
- Sample PES statement: Undesirable food choices related to client now eating most meals in college cafeteria as evidenced by inability to select foods consistent with nutrition education for CKD stage 5 predialysis.

Source: Data are from reference 1.

Figure 3.1 Common Nutrition Diagnoses in My Practice

Nutrition Diagnosis	Definition	Etiologies	Signs and Symptoms	Sample PES Statements
1.				
2.				
3.				
4.				

NUTRITION DIAGNOSIS REFERENCE SHEET

RDs may want to create their own reference sheet that lists the nutrition diagnoses they use most often and sample PES statements. Figure 3.1 presents an example of a chart that can be completed and used when needed. For each nutrition diagnosis, take care to use the exact IDNT nutrition diagnosis label and definition and write one or two sample PES statements based on your own patients/clients.

CASE STUDY—NCP STEP 2: DIAGNOSIS

Full nutrition assessment data for this case study of a 56-year-old Cambodian woman with ESRD are presented at the end of Chapter 2. The following sections present some possible nutrition diagnoses and related PES statements. Later chapters continue to develop the case study with information appropriate to subsequent steps in the NCP.

Intake Domain

- Nutrition diagnosis: Excessive carbohydrate intake.
- Sample PES statement: Excessive carbohydrate intake related to cultural food patterns and consumption of carbonated colas as evidenced by food recall and by patient reports of drinking regular cola to treat nausea.

Clinical Domain

- Nutrition diagnosis: Altered nutrition-related laboratory values (serum phosphorus).
- Sample PES statements:

- Altered nutrition-related laboratory values (serum phosphorus) related to missed binder doses prior to admission as evidenced by patient report and by serum phosphorus of 5.7 mg/dL.
- Altered nutrition-related laboratory values (serum albumin) related to altered nutrient utilization in inflammatory state as evidenced by serum albumin of 1.6 g/dL in a patient with acute peritonitis.

Behavioral-Environmental Domain

- Nutrition diagnosis: Limited adherence to nutrition-related recommendations.
- Sample PES statement: Limited adherence to nutrition-related recommendations related to the use of carbonated beverages to treat GI symptoms as evidenced by patient reports of drinking cola beverages during episodes of nausea and vomiting.

Chapter 4

Nutrition Intervention— Part One: Planning the Nutrition Prescription

Nutrition intervention is the third step of the Nutrition Care Process (NCP). As stated in the *IDNT Reference Manual* (1), the goal of nutrition intervention is "to resolve or improve the identified nutrition problem by planning and implementing appropriate nutrition interventions that are tailored to the patient's/client's needs." Furthermore, "the selection of nutrition intervention is driven by the nutrition diagnosis and its etiology," which are identified in the PES (ie, problem, etiology, and signs and symptoms) statement (see Chapter 3 of this guide).

The nutrition prescription is defined as "the patient's/client's recommended dietary intake of energy and/or selected foods or nutrients based on current reference standards and dietary guidelines and the patient's/client's health condition and nutrition diagnosis" (1). The purpose of the nutrition prescription is to communicate the dietetics practitioner's diet/nutrition recommendation based on the nutrition assessment (1).

Nutrition prescription recommendations in this chapter are based on the recognized practice guidelines described in Chapter 1 (see Box 4.1) (1). Chapter 5 covers implementation of the nutrition prescription.

Box 4.1   Considerations in Developing a Nutrition Prescription for Chronic Kidney Disease (CKD)

The nutrition intervention includes developing the nutrition prescription by evaluating:

- Energy needs based on nutrition assessment and diagnosis (eg, kcal/kg/d)
- Carbohydrate distribution to balance estimated calorie and protein needs
- Protein needs based on stage of CKD and treatment (eg, conservative management of renal disease vs renal replacement therapy) to promote normal nutritional status
- Fat distribution to balance energy and protein needs and promote heart health
- Vitamin intake (eg, over-the-counter [OTC] supplements, fortified foods) regarding vitamins pertinent to CKD, including vitamin C, vitamin D, and others as appropriate
- Mineral intake (eg, OTC supplements, fortified foods) regarding minerals pertinent to CKD, including calcium, iron, phosphorus, potassium, sodium, and others as appropriate
- Fluid intake based on fluid balance
- Fiber intake
- Level of bioactive substances
- Enteral or parenteral nutrition as appropriate
- Modification of texture and/or liquid consistency
- Renal diet exchanges, for each food group, to meet energy, protein, carbohydrate, fat, vitamin, and mineral needs

Source: Data are from reference 1.

PLANNING THE NUTRITION PRESCRIPTION: CKD STAGES 3 TO 5 (NOT ON DIALYSIS)

Table 4.1 (2,4,9,29,30) summarizes medical nutrition therapy (MNT) goals for patients/clients with chronic kidney disease (CKD) stages 1 through 5 (nondialysis). Table 4.2 (3,4,9,29) offers recommendations for lipid treatment goals for the same patient/client population. The following sections provide additional information on specific nutrient requirements for patients/clients with CKD stages 3 through 5 (not on dialysis) as well as the use of nutrition support.

Table 4.1 MNT Recommendations for Chronic Kidney Disease (CKD) Stages 1 Through 5, Nondialysis, With or Without Diabetes

Nutrient	Recommendations (References)
Energy, kcal/kg	Stages 1–5: 23–35 (2)
Sodium, g/d	Stages 1–5: <2.4 (2)
Phosphorus, mg/d	Stages 1–2: 1,700 (2) Stages 3–5: 800–1,000 (2,30)
Calcium, g/d	Stages 1–2: N/A Stages 3–5: ≤2 (1.5 g/d from binders in CKD stage 5) (30)
Potassium, g/d	Stages 1–2: >4 (4) Stages 3–5: 2.4 (2,4)
Protein, g/kg/d	Stages 1–2: no diabetes 1.4 (4) Stages 3–5, no diabetes: 0.6–0.8; with diabetes: 0.8–0.9 (2)
Carbohydrate, % of calories	Stages 1–4: 50%–60% (4)
Fiber, g/d	Stages 1–5: 20–30 (9)
Soluble fiber, g/d	Stages 1–5: 5–10 (9)
Cholesterol, mg/d	Stages 1–4: <200 (4)

(continued)

Table 4.1   MNT Recommendations for Chronic Kidney Disease (CKD) Stages 1 Through 5, Nondialysis, With or Without Diabetes (continued)

Nutrient	Recommendations (References)
Total fat,[a] % of calories	Stages 1–4: <30% (4)
Saturated fat, % of calories	Stages 1–4: <10% (4)
PUFA, % of calories	Stages 1–5: ≤10% (9)
MUFA, % of calories	Stages 1–5: ≤ 20% (9)
Trans fat	Minimal intake (29)

Abbreviations: N/A, information not available (no evidence-based standard has been published); PUFA, polyunsaturated fatty acids; MUFA, monounsaturated fatty acids.

[a]Adjust so total calories from protein, fat, and carbohydrate are 100%. Emphasize such whole-food sources as fresh vegetables, whole grains, nuts, legumes, low-fat or nonfat dairy products, canola oil, olive oil, cold-water fish, and poultry (2).

Source: Data are from references 2, 4, 9, 29, and 30.

Table 4.2   Lipid Treatment Goals in Chronic Kidney Disease (CKD) Stages 1 Through 5, not on Dialysis[a]

Lipid Panel	Lipid Treatment Goals (References)
Total cholesterol	150–180 mg/dL (3)
HDL	Men: ≥40 mg/dL (29) Women: ≥50 mg/dL (29)
Triglycerides (TG)	<200 mg/dL (9)
LDL	<100 mg/dL (4,9,29) <70 mg/dL may be recommended for patients with diabetes (29)
non-HDL[b]	<130 mg/dL (for patients with TG ≥200) (9)

[a]Recheck lipid panels annually or 2–3 months after change in treatment or clinical status (eg, a change in albuminuria/proteinuria or GFR).

[b]non-HDL = Total cholesterol – HDL

Source: Data are from references 3, 4, 9, and 29.

Protein Prescription

CKD Without Diabetes and with an eGFR less than 50 mL/min/1.73m²

For adults with CKD without diabetes, not on dialysis, with an eGFR less than 50 mL/min/1.73m², the RD should recommend or prescribe a protein-controlled diet providing 0.6 to 0.8 g dietary protein per kg of body weight per day (see Table 4.1). When recommending lower protein intakes, the RD should use clinical judgment and consider the patient's/client's level of motivation, willingness to participate in frequent follow-up, and risk for protein-energy malnutrition. Protein-restricted diets (0.7 g dietary protein per kg of body weight per day, ensuring adequate caloric intake) can slow GFR decline and maintain stable nutritional status in adult nondiabetic patients/clients with CKD (2).

Protein Intake for Diabetic Nephropathy

For patients/clients with diabetic nephropathy, the RD should recommend or prescribe a protein-controlled diet providing 0.8 to 0.9 g of protein per kg of body weight per day (see Table 4.1). Dietary protein provided at a level of 0.7 g per kg of body weight per day may result in hypoalbuminemia. Research indicates protein-restricted diets improve microalbuminuria (2).

Very Low–Protein Intake (in International Settings)

A very low–protein diet may be considered for patients/clients in international settings where keto-acid analogs are available. For adults with CKD without diabetes, not on dialysis, with an eGFR less than 20mL/min/1.73m², a very low–protein diet that provides 0.3 to 0.5 g dietary protein per kg of body weight per day *plus* keto-acid analogs (to meet estimated protein needs) may be recommended. To maintain adequate nutritional status for patients/clients with CKD who consume a very low–protein controlled diet (0.3 to 0.5 g/kg/d), additional keto-acid analogs and vitamin or mineral supplementation are needed (2).

Energy Prescription

It is important to use clinical judgment to determine the ideal edema-free body weight to use to calculate energy needs for patients/clients with CKD (2). See Chapter 2 for a full discussion of how to determine the appropriate weight for energy calculations.

For adults with CKD, the RD should recommend an energy intake between 23 and 35 kcal/kg/d, based on the following factors (see Table 4.1):

- Weight status and goals
- Age and gender
- Level of physical activity
- Metabolic stressors

Research indicates that energy intakes between 23 and 35 kcal/kg/d are adequate to prevent malnutrition in adults with CKD (2).

Once daily energy needs are determined, it is imperative to balance the intake of protein, carbohydrate, and fat to promote a healthful diet that does not include an excessive amount of any specific macronutrient.

Carbohydrate Prescription

Diabetes is the leading cause of CKD in developed countries, and it is becoming the major cause of CKD in developing countries as the incidence of both diabetes and obesity increases (4). Intensive treatment of hyperglycemia that avoids hypoglycemia can prevent diabetic kidney disease (DKD) and may slow the progression of established kidney disease (2).

For adults with diabetes and CKD, the RD should implement MNT for diabetes care to manage hyperglycemia and to achieve a target Hgb A1c of approximately 7% (2,11). Patients/clients with advanced cardiovascular disease and an Hgb A1c less than 6.5% may have an increased mortality risk (2).

For CKD patients/clients with diabetes, consider limiting intake of dietary carbohydrate to 50% to 60% of calories per day (see Table 4.1) (4). The dietary carbohydrate and fat recommendation must provide adequate calories to spare dietary protein for anabolism and to achieve and maintain a healthy weight.

Fat Prescription

The National Kidney Foundation considers individuals with renal disease to have a risk of heart disease equal to the risk of those with confirmed coronary heart disease (9). Therefore, the fat prescription should set healthful targets for the amounts and types of fat consumed (ie, saturated, *trans,* polyunsaturated, and monounsaturated fats). To achieve lipid treatment goals (Table 4.2), daily total dietary fat and saturated fat intake should be limited to less than 30% and 10% of calories, respectively (see Table 4.1) (4).

According to the Evidence-Based Nutrition Practice Guidelines for Chronic Kidney Disease, "there is insufficient evidence to support fish oil therapy to improve renal function…or graft survival for kidney transplant patients/ clients" (2). However, evidence suggests that fish oil supplementation may be beneficial in reducing oxidative stress and improving lipid profiles in adults with CKD (2).

Vitamin Prescription

- Vitamin A supplementation is not recommended in CKD Stages 3 to 5 because serum vitamin A levels may increase as renal function worsens (see Table 4.3) (31).

- Vitamin D supplementation is recommended if a patient's/client's serum level of 25-hydroxyvitamin D is less than 30 ng/mL (2). Recent literature recommends 800 to 1,000 IU of cholecalciferol (D-3) per day (see Table 4.3) (31).

- Vitamin C supplementation is sometimes used to improve iron absorption in adults with CKD and iron-deficiency anemia (2). Daily vitamin C intake should be restricted to an upper limit of 60 mg/d (see Table 4.3) (31). Patients/clients with CKD are at risk of hyperoxalosis at higher vitamin C doses (2).

- For adults with CKD and elevated MCV, the RD should evaluate vitamin B-12 and folic acid levels and recommend supplementation as needed. A dietary protein restriction (≤ 0.6 g/kg/d) may contribute to vitamin B-12 deficiency. CKD patients/clients have a predisposition for anemia, and all potential causes should be investigated (2).

- The RD should recommend a multivitamin preparation sufficient to maintain indices of adequate nutritional status to adults with CKD who are not on dialysis and have no known nutrient deficiency (biochemical or physical) if they could be at higher nutritional risk due to poor dietary intake and decreasing GFR (2).

- No peer-reviewed research has reported the effects of micronutrients on preserving kidney function among nondialyzed adults with CKD, nephrotic syndrome, diabetic nephropathy, or kidney transplant (2).

Table 4.3   Recommended Vitamin Supplementation for Patients/Clients with Chronic Kidney Disease (CKD), not on Dialysis

Vitamin	Daily Recommendations[a]
Vitamin A	Supplementation is not recommended
Vitamin D	800–1,000 IU
Vitamin E	15 mg
Vitamin K	Men: 120 mcg Women: 90 mcg
Vitamin C	30–60 mg
Thiamin (vitamin B-1)	Men, ages 50–70 y: 1.2 mg Women, ages 50–70 y: 1.1 mg
Riboflavin (vitamin B-2)	Men: 1.3 mg Women: 1.1 mg
Niacin (vitamin B-3)	Men: 16 mg Women: 14 mg
Pyridoxine (vitamin B-6)	5 mg
Folic acid	Intake should be adequate; no supplement needed
Cobalamin (vitamin B-12)	No supplement needed unless protein intake is ≤0.6 g/kg/d
Pantothenic acid (vitamin B-5)	Age >51 y: 5 mg = Adequate Intake

[a]Recommendations are for both men and women unless otherwise specified.
Source: Data are from reference 31.

Electrolyte and Mineral Prescription

Sodium

Limiting sodium intake to less than 2.4 g/d is recommended for patients/clients with CKD stages 3 to 5. This goal should be adjusted as appropriate based on a patient's/client's fluid balance, blood pressure control, and other clinical findings (2).

Potassium

When a patient/client with CKD stages 3 to 5 has hyperkalemia, the RD should recommend a potassium intake of less than 2.4 g/d and consider relevant clinical factors, including serum potassium levels, medications that may affect potassium, glycemic control, and other issues (2). Hypokalemia or hyperkalemia can have a direct effect on cardiac function, with potential for cardiac arrhythmia and sudden death (2).

Calcium

For adults with CKD stages 3 to 5, the RD should recommend a total elemental calcium intake (including dietary calcium, calcium supplementation, and calcium-based phosphate binders) of 2,000 mg/d or less. CKD patients/clients have a predisposition for mineral and bone disorders. Serum calcium concentration is an important factor in regulating PTH secretion and therefore affects bone integrity and soft-tissue calcification (2). The RD should be aware of the risks of hypercalcemia, including soft-tissue calcification (2).

Phosphorus

Hyperphosphatemia and its associated conditions begin when GFR is less than 60 mL/min/1.73 m^2 (2). Because MBD is common in CKD, phosphorus control is essential for the treatment and prevention of secondary hyperparathyroidism, renal bone disease, and soft-tissue calcification (2).

For adults with elevated serum phosphorus levels as well as CKD stages 3 to 5, the RD should recommend a low-phosphorus diet with 800 to 1,000 mg of dietary phosphorus per day (or 10 to 12 mg phosphorus per gram of protein per day) (2).

For adults with CKD stages 3 to 5, the dose and timing of phosphate binders should be individually adjusted to the phosphate content of meals and snacks to achieve desired serum phosphorus levels. Serum phosphorus levels are difficult to control with dietary restrictions alone (2). Treatment to manage serum phosphorus needs to be individualized and may include dietary phosphate restriction, phosphate binders, calcium and vitamin D supplementation, and self-management training (2).

Aluminum

Aluminum-containing antacid medications (eg, aluminum hydroxide) may cause blood/serum levels of aluminum to rise in patients/clients with CKD (32).

Iron

When adults with CKD have serum ferritin levels less than 500 ng/mL and their percent serum transferrin saturation (TSAT) is less than 30%, oral or intravenous iron supplementation may be recommended. The amount of iron supplementation recommended should maintain levels of serum iron that will adequately support erythropoiesis (2,33).

Iron absorption may be impaired by other medications, such as phosphate binders (2).

Magnesium

There are no evidenced-based guidelines that evaluate the appropriate daily intake of magnesium for patients/clients with CKD (2). The RD should recognize that magnesium-containing antacid medications (eg, Maalox and milk of magnesia) may cause blood/serum levels of magnesium to rise in patients/clients with CKD (32).

Enteral Nutrition Prescription

Patients/clients with renal failure who require nutrition support therapy should receive enteral nutrition if their intestinal function permits it (14). Macronutrient, vitamin, and mineral guidelines for CKD apply to the prescription for an enteral solution. The patient's/client's serum concentrations of potassium, magnesium, phosphorus, and calcium should be monitored so electrolyte intake can be adjusted appropriately (14).

Parenteral Nutrition Prescription

If altered gastrointestinal function prevents the patient/client from taking enteral nutrition, parenteral nutrition should be considered to support nutritional status. Tables 4.4 and 4.5 (34) and Box 4.2 (35) provide examples of formulas and compositions that may be used for these patients/clients.

Table 4.4   Sample Parenteral Nutrition Formulations

	PPN	Standard TPN	Concentrated TPN
Carbohydrate,[a] g/L	100	200	200
Amino acids,[b] g/L	35	50	75
Electrolytes	Adjust per metabolic profile	Adjust per metabolic profile	Adjust per metabolic profile

Abbreviations: PPN, peripheral parenteral nutrition; TPN, total parenteral nutrition
[a]Carbohydrate: 3.4 kcal/g.
[b]Amino acids: 4 kcal/g.
Source: Data are from reference 34.

Table 4.5   Sample Lipid Formulations for Parenteral Nutrition

Lipid Concentration	Volume, mL	Energy, kcal/mL	Total Energy, kcal
10% lipids	500	1.1	550
20% lipids	250	2.0	500
20% lipids	500	2.0	1,000

Source: Data are from reference 34.

Box 4.2   Suggested Composition of Parenteral Nutrition Solution for Adults with Chronic Kidney Disease (CKD)

Macronutrients, Fluid, and Electrolytes
- Energy: 25–35 kcal/kg/d[a]
- Amino acids (mixture of essential and nonessential amino acids):
  - Predialysis: 0.6–1 g/kg/d
  - Chronic dialysis: 1.2–1.3 g/kg/d
  - CRRT: ≥1 g/kg/d
- Dextrose: Consider all sources of dextrose (intravenous fluids, dialytic therapy).
- Lipids:
  - <1 g/kg/d or 20%–30% of total calories
  - Include propofol infusion in lipid sources
  - PPN lipid content should not exceed 60% of total calories
- Fluid: Volume depends on patient's/client's tolerance and requirements.
- Electrolytes: Amounts vary according to patient's/client's tolerance. Higher requirements may occur with CRRT.

Minerals
- Sodium: 40–60 mEq/L (920–1,380 mg/L)
- Potassium: 10–40 mEq/L (390–1,560 mg/L)
- Phosphorus: 5–10 mmol/L
- Calcium[b]: 5–10 mEq/L
- Magnesium: 5–10 mEq/L (120–240 mg/L)
- Chloride and acetate: Proportions vary depending on acid-base status.

(continued)

**Box 4.2   Suggested Composition of Parenteral Nutrition
Solution for Adults with Chronic Kidney Disease (CKD)**
(continued)

Vitamins
- Vitamin A: 3,300 IU/d
- Vitamin D: 200 IU/d
- Vitamin E: 10 IU/d
- Vitamin K: 150 mcg/d
- Vitamin C: 200 mg/d (IHD: 100 mg/d)
- Thiamin (B-1): 6 mg/d
- Riboflavin (B-2): 3.6 mg/d
- Niacin (B-3): 40 mg/d
- Pyridoxine (B-6): 6 mg/d
- Cobalamin (B-12): 5 mcg/d
- Folate: 600 mcg/d
- Pantothenic acid (B-5): 15 mg/d
- Biotin: 60 mcg/d

Trace Elements
- Zinc: 2.5–4 mg/d
- Copper: 0.5–1.5 mg/d
- Chromium: 10–15 mcg/d
- Manganese: 0.15–0.8 mg/d
- Selenium: 40–120 mcg/d

Abbreviations: CRRT, continuous renal replacement therapy; PPN, peripheral parenteral nutrition; IHD, intermittent hemodialysis.
[a]Use estimated edema-free body weight.
[b]Calcium citrate is not recommended as it enhances aluminum absorption (24).
Source: Adapted with permission from reference 35: Byham–Gray L, Wiesen K, Stover J. *A Clinical Guide To Nutrition Care In Kidney Disease.* 2nd ed. Chicago, IL: Academy of Nutrition and Dietetics; 2013.

PLANNING THE NUTRITION PRESCRIPTION: HEMODIALYSIS AND PERITONEAL DIALYSIS

Table 4.6 summarizes MNT recommendations for patients/clients on hemodialysis (HD) or peritoneal dialysis (PD) (3,16,24,30,36). The following sections provide additional information about specific nutrient requirements as well as the use of nutrition support.

Table 4.6   Hemodialysis and Peritoneal Dialysis Medical Nutrition Therapy Recommendations

Nutrients	Recommendations (References)
Energy	Age <60 y, HD or PD: 35 kcal/kg (3,16) Age ≥60 y, HD or PD: 30–35 kcal/kg (3,36)
Protein	HD: ≥1.1 g/kg; ≥50% HBV (3,16) PD: ≥1.2–1.3 g/kg; ≥50% HBV (3,36)
Carbohydrate, total fat, and saturated fat	HD or PD: Promote glycemic and lipid control
Potassium	HD: 50–70 mEq/d (16) PD: Restricted with hyperkalemia (24)
Sodium	HD: 2–2.3 g/d (16) PD: N/A
Calcium	HD or PD: ≤2 g/d total, with ≤1.5 g/d from binders (30)
Phosphorus	HD or PD: 800–1,000 mg/d (30)
Vitamin D	HD or PD: Supplement if patient/client has deficiency and when CKD-MBD lab values are at target (30)
Multivitamin supplement	HD: see Table 4.8 (16) PD: N/A
Fluid	HD: IDWG 4%–4.5% dry weight (16) PD: Maintain edema-free weight (24)
Fiber	HD or PD: 20–25 g/d (24)

Abbreviations: HD, hemodialysis; PD, peritoneal dialysis; HBV, high biological value; N/A, not available (ie, evidence-based guidelines have not been established for this topic); IDWG, interdialytic weight gain; CKD-MBD, chronic kidney disease–mineral and bone disorder.

Source: Data are from references 3, 16, 24, 30, and 36.

Protein Prescription

For patients/clients on HD or PD, at least 50% of the protein should be from sources of high biological value (HBV) (3).

Hemodialysis

For clinically stable maintenance HD patients/clients, KDOQI recommends a protein intake of 1.2 g/kg/d (3). The European Best Practice Guidelines (EBPG) recommend at least 1.1 g/kg/d for HD patients/clients but otherwise make protein recommendations similar to those in KDOQI (16).

The optimum protein intake for a patient/client on maintenance dialysis who is acutely ill is at least 1.2 to 1.3 g/kg/d (3).

Peritoneal Dialysis

For stable PD patients/clients, 1.2 to 1.3 g protein per kg per day are recommended (3). RDs should use clinical judgment to evaluate whether patients/clients with peritonitis, malnutrition, or other metabolic stress need increased amounts of dietary protein (35).

Energy Prescription

The dialysis patient/client should be prescribed an edema-free body weight or estimated dry weight. This weight prescription may be based on clinical findings (such as blood pressure, weight gain between treatments, and symptoms such as headaches or cramps), bioimpedance measurements, or continuous blood volume monitoring, or it may be determined using other assessment tools (37,38). This dry weight represents the patient's/client's target weight after a dialysis treatment, and it may be used for calculations of energy needs in HD and PD.

The KDOQI recommended daily energy intake for maintenance HD or chronic PD patients/clients younger than 60 years of age is 35 kcal/kg/d, and the recommended daily energy intake for maintenance HD or chronic PD patients/clients 60 years or older is 30 to 35 kcal/kg/d (3). The EBPG suggest up to 40 kcal/kg/d for HD patients/clients but otherwise provide energy recommendations similar to those from KDOQI (16). In acute illness, the KDOQI energy recommendations are considered minimum energy goals (3). Please see Chapter 2 (Tables 2.3 to 2.6 and Box 2.9) regarding the appropriate weight for nutrient calculations.

For patients/clients receiving PD, it is also necessary to adjust the energy prescription to allow for the energy absorbed from the dialysate (Table 4.7) (24).

Table 4.7   Dextrose Concentrations of Peritoneal Dialysis Solutions

	1 Liter	*2 Liters*	*2.5 Liters*	*3 Liters*
1.5% dextrose	15 g[a]	30 g[a]	45 g[a]	60 g[a]
2.5% dextrose	25 g[a]	50 g[a]	62.5 g[a]	75 g[a]
4.25% dextrose	42.5 g[a]	85g[a]	106.25 g[a]	127.5 g[a]

Percentage of dextrose absorption (see sample calculation in case study at the end of this chapter): Continuous ambulatory peritoneal dialysis (CAPD) = 60%–70% dextrose absorption; continuous cyclic peritoneal dialysis (CCPD) = 40%–50% dextrose absorption.

[a] 3.4 kcal per g dextrose

Source: Adapted from reference 24: McCann L, ed. *Pocket Guide to Nutrition Assessment of the Patient with Chronic Kidney Disease.* 4th ed. New York, NY: National Kidney Foundation; 2009. Adapted with permission from National Kidney Foundation, Inc.

Carbohydrate Prescription

In the renal diet, carbohydrate and fat should deliver adequate energy to ensure that protein is used for physiologic functions (4). Carbohydrate intake needs to be sufficient without being excessive (4). Although the protein provided by carbohydrate foods is not of high biological value (HBV), it needs to be included in the total daily protein calculations for the renal diet (35).

The dextrose provided by the peritoneal dialysate solution must be considered when managing blood glucose control for patients/clients with diabetes who are receiving PD. To prevent unwanted weight gain and to optimize diabetic control, peritoneal dialysis exchanges should be done with the lowest dextrose solutions that provide effective dialysis adequacy. To prevent unwanted weight gain, subtract the calories provided by PD exchanges from the patient's/client's estimated total daily calorie requirements.

Fat Prescription

When developing a nutrition prescription, the RD must consider the high cardiovascular disease risk profile of patients/clients with CKD (9). The fat prescription should set healthful targets for the amounts and types of fat to be consumed (ie, saturated, *trans*, polyunsaturated, and monounsaturated fats), with the goal of improving the patient's/client's lipid profile.

Vitamin Prescription

Most expert guidelines, with the exception of the EBPG (16), do not include recommendations for dialysis patients/clients about the intake of vitamins other than vitamin D. However, it is recommended that dialysis patients/clients take a renal multivitamin daily to replace water-soluble vitamins that are lost with the dialysis process (16). Vitamin recommendations for different situations are included in Table 4.8 (16) and Box 4.3 (10). Use professional judgment regarding supplementation in cases of malabsorption or vitamin deficiency.

Table 4.8   Daily Vitamin Recommendations for Hemodialysis

Vitamin	Recommendation
Vitamin A	Intake: 700–900 mcg; supplement not recommended
Vitamin D	Adjust dose based on phosphorus, calcium, iPTH levels
Vitamin E	Supplement: 400–800 IU
Vitamin K	Intake: 90–120 mcg; supplement not recommended
Vitamin C	Supplement: 75–90 mg
Thiamin (vitamin B-1)	Supplement: 1.1–1.2 mg
Riboflavin (vitamin B-2)	Supplement: 1.1–1.3 mg
Niacin (vitamin B-3)	Supplement: 14–16 mg
Pyridoxine (vitamin B-6)	Supplement: 10 mg
Folic acid	Supplement: 1 mg
Cobalamin (vitamin B-12)	Supplement: 2.4 mcg
Pantothenic acid (vitamin B-5)	Supplement: 5 mg
Biotin	Supplement: 30 mcg

Source: Data are from reference 16.

Box 4.3   KDIGO Recommendations for Calcitriol, Vitamin D Analogs, and Calcimimetics in Chronic Kidney Disease (CKD) Stage 5D

- In patients with CKD stage 5D and elevated or rising PTH, we [KDIGO] suggest calcitriol, or vitamin D analogs, or calcimimetics, or a combination of calcimimetics and calcitriol or vitamin D analogs be used to lower PTH (2B).
- It is reasonable that the initial drug selection for the treatment of elevated PTH be based on serum calcium and phosphorus levels and other aspects of CKD-MBD (not graded).
- It is reasonable that calcium or non-calcium-based phosphate binder dosage be adjusted so that treatments to control PTH do not compromise levels of phosphorus and calcium (not graded).

(continued)

Box 4.3   KDIGO Recommendations for Calcitriol, Vitamin D Analogs, and Calcimimetics in Chronic Kidney Disease (CKD) Stage 5D (continued)

- We recommend that, in patients with hypercalcemia, calcitriol or another vitamin D sterol be reduced or stopped (1B).
- We suggest that, in patients with hyperphosphatemia, calcitriol or another vitamin D sterol be reduced or stopped (2D).
- We suggest that, in patients with hypocalcemia, calcimimetics be reduced or stopped depending on severity, concomitant medications, and clinical signs and symptoms (2D).
- We suggest that, if the intact PTH levels fall below two times the upper limit of normal for the assay, calcitriol, vitamin D analogs, and/or calcimimetics be reduced or stopped (2C).

Key to strength of recommendation: 1 = strong evidence; 2 = weak evidence. Quality of Evidence: A = high; B = moderate; C = low; D = very low. *Source:* Reprinted from reference 10: Kidney Disease: Improving Global Outcomes (KDIGO) CKD-MBD Work Group. KDIGO clinical practice guidelines for the diagnosis, evaluation, prevention, and treatment of chronic kidney disease-mineral and bone disorder (CKD-MBD). *Kidney Int.* 2009; 76 (suppl 113):S1–S130. www.kdigo.org/clinical_practice_guidelines/kdigo _guideline_for_ckd-mbd.php. Reprinted with permission from National Kidney Foundation, Inc.

Electrolyte and Mineral Prescription

Sodium

Intake should be limited to 2,000 to 2,300 mg sodium per day to control fluid gain and blood pressure (16).

Potassium

According to the EBPG, dietary potassium intake should be limited to 1,950 to 2,730 mg/d (50 to 70 mEq/d) to maintain serum potassium levels of less than 6 mEq/L (16).

Calcium

Because of the danger of hypercalcemia and tissue calcification, elemental calcium intake should not exceed 2,000 mg/d (16,30). The elemental calcium provided by calcium-based phosphorus binders should not provide more than 1,500 mg calcium per day (16,30).

Phosphorus

Daily intake of 800 to 1,000 mg phosphate is recommended. However, dietary phosphorus control should not compromise protein intake (16). See Box 4.4 for KDIGO recommendations (10).

Box 4.4   KDIGO Recommendations for Phosphorus Control in Chronic Kidney Disease (CKD) Stage 5D

- Treatment should reduce "elevated phosphorus…toward the normal range (2C)."
- Maintain "serum calcium in the normal range (2D)."
- Use phosphate-binding agents to control hyperphosphatemia (2B). Evaluate the stage of CKD, "presence of other components of CKD-MBD, concomitant therapies, and side-effect profile" of the selected binder (not graded).
- In patients/clients with hyperphosphatemia, "calcium-based phosphorus binders and/or the dose of calcitriol or vitamin D analog" should be limited when there is "persistent or recurrent hypercalcemia (1B)." Use of calcium-based phosphate binders should be limited when there is "arterial calcification (2C), and/or adynamic bone disease (2C), and/or if serum PTH levels are persistently low (2C)."
- Hyperphosphatemia should be treated by "limiting dietary phosphorus…in combination with other treatments (2D)."

Key to strength of recommendation: 1 = strong evidence; 2 = weak evidence. Quality of Evidence: A = high; B = moderate; C = low; D = very low. *Source:* Data are from reference 10.

Aluminum

The kidneys are involved in the excretion of aluminum, and aluminum can accumulate in the bodies of adults with CKD (30). Therefore, long-term use of aluminum-containing phosphorus binders "should be avoided to prevent aluminum intoxication" (10). For this reason, use of aluminum-based phosphate binders (ie, aluminum hydroxide) by adults should be limited to 4 weeks or less and reserved for only those times when the serum phosphorus level is greater than 7 mg/dL (30).

Iron

The recommended daily intake of iron is 8 mg for men and 15 mg for women (16). When a patient/client receives an erythropoiesis-stimulating agent (ESA), additional supplementary oral iron is appropriate (unless the patient/client is receiving iron intravenously) to maintain adequate serum transferrin and serum ferritin levels and to achieve a target hemoglobin concentration of 9 to 11.5 g/dL (33). To improve iron absorption, oral iron supplements should be taken between meals and not with phosphorus binders (16).

Magnesium

There are no evidenced-based guidelines that evaluate the appropriate daily intake of magnesium in CKD. Magnesium-containing antacid medications (eg, Maalox, milk of magnesia) may cause blood/serum levels of magnesium to rise in CKD (32).

Zinc

Daily nutritional intake of 8 to 12 mg of elemental zinc for women and 10 to 15 mg for men is recommended.

However, routine zinc supplementation in the absence of biochemical confirmation of a deficiency is not recommended. When a patient's/client's zinc intake is chronically inadequate and the patient/client has symptoms of zinc deficiency (impaired taste or smell, skin fragility, impotence, or peripheral neuropathy), daily supplementation with 50 mg of elemental zinc may be considered for 3 to 6 months. At that time, biochemical levels should be rechecked and zinc supplementation should be discontinued if serum levels have normalized (16).

Selenium

Daily intake of 55 mcg of selenium is appropriate, but routine selenium supplementation is not recommended. It may be appropriate for hemodialysis patients/clients with symptoms of selenium deficiency (such as cardiomyopathy, skeletal myopathy, thyroid dysfunction, hemolysis, or dermatosis) to take selenium supplements for 3 to 6 months (16).

Fluid Prescription

Current fluid intake guidelines for maintenance HD patients/clients vary from 500 to 1,000 mL/d plus urine output (16). In general, achievement of this goal will support an interdialytic weight gain of 2 to 2.5 kg (16).

Enteral Nutrition Prescription

When a patient's/client's oral intake is not meeting minimum nutrient recommendations, nutritional supplements that are specifically formulated for people on dialysis should be prescribed (3,16). If tube feeding is required, the general nutrition recommendations for dialysis patients/clients will apply to the enteral nutrition prescription.

Box 5.1 in Chapter 5 lists a selection of available enteral formulas.

Parenteral Nutrition Prescription
(Including Use of Intradialytic Parenteral Nutrition)

When altered gastrointestinal function makes the use of enteral nutrition impossible, parenteral nutrition to meet 100% of estimated needs is recommended (14).

Unique to dialysis is the ability to provide intra-dialytic parenteral nutrition (IDPN) (Boxes 4.5 and 4.6) (24,35,39). Three expert groups have published differing recommendations regarding IDPN:

- According to KDOQI, IDPN should be considered if it is needed in addition to oral intake to satisfy protein and energy requirements (3).
- The EBPG recommends IDPN in malnourished patients/clients only if their daily spontaneous nutrient intake is greater than 20 kcal per kilogram of IBW and greater than 0.8 g protein per kilogram of IBW. Otherwise, total parenteral nutrition (TPN) infused over the entire day is indicated (16).
- A.S.P.E.N. suggests that IDPN should not be used as a nutritional supplement in malnourished hemo-dialysis patients/clients in the United States (14). Findings from peer-reviewed research were inconsistent regarding the benefit of IDPN. A.S.P.E.N. has concluded that available research does not offer strong support for IDPN and has called for further research to evaluate potential clinical advantages (14).

Box 4.5   Macronutrient and Electrolyte Considerations in Intradialytic Parenteral Nutrition (IDPN)

Amino Acids (AA)
- IDPN should contain essential and nonessential AA (35).
- To limit IDPN complications, current formulations provide higher protein concentrations with modest amounts of dextrose and lipid in volumes below 1 liter (35).
- Recommend 1.2–1.4 g AA per kg of body weight (24,35).
- To avoid acidosis, monitor serum bicarbonate levels (24).

Dextrose
- Check peripheral glucose 1 hour before IDPN, at least once 1 hour into an infusion, and 1 hour after an infusion of IDPN (24,35).
- To improve glycemic control, the recommended amount of dextrose per bag of IDPN is 45–75 g (35).
- Consider providing a snack ½ hour before an IDPN treatment is completed to combat potential hypoglycemia (24,35).
- Recommend 5–8 units of insulin per 1,000 mL IDPN when blood glucose level is >300 mg/dL (35).
- Tight glycemic control has not been studied in patients/clients receiving IDPN but may not be appropriate due to the hazards of hypoglycemia. Increasing insulin by 2 units per treatment to reach an acceptable level of blood glucose control, usually <200 mg/dL, may be recommended (35).

Lipids
- Limit lipid delivery to ≤2.5 g/kg/d or ≤60% of total calories (39).
- Check serum triglycerides prior to first two IDPN treatments; continue to recheck every month (35). Some experts recommend limiting lipids to ≤2 mg/kg/min if triglycerides >300 mg/dL (24) and holding lipids if triglycerides >400 mg/dL, as such data suggest that lipids are not being well cleared (24,35).
- Avoid lipids when the patient/client is allergic to egg and/or soy (24).

(continued)

Box 4.5   **Macronutrient and Electrolyte Considerations in Intradialytic Parenteral Nutrition (IDPN)** (continued)

Lipids (continued)
- May suggest omitting lipids in the first 1 to 4 weeks of IDPN to allow patient/client to adjust to the dextrose and AA infusion without any confounding side effects from lipids (35).

Electrolytes
- Intracellular shifts of electrolytes can result from the glucose infusion (35). Monitor potassium, calcium, phosphorus, and magnesium levels at each dialysis treatment until they are stable; then check them monthly (35).

Source: Data are from references 24, 35, and 39.

Box 4.6   **Intradialytic Parenteral Nutrition (IDPN) Formulas: Examples for a 70-kg Patient**

High-Dextrose, High-Calorie, and High-Volume Formula
- Dextrose[a]: 125 g D_{70} (179 mL, 425 kcal)
- 1.3 g amino acids (AA)/kg: 90 g of 15% AA (600 mL, 360 kcal)
- 20% lipids[b] (optional): 30 g (150 mL, 300 kcal)
- Total volume: 779 mL (929 mL with optional lipids)
- Total energy: 785 kcal (1,085 kcal with optional lipids)

Moderate-Dextrose, Moderate-Calorie, and Moderate-Volume Formula
- Dextrose[a]: 75 g D_{70} (107 mL, 255 kcal)
- 1.3 g AA/kg: 90 g of 15% AA (600 mL, 360 kcal)
- 20% lipids[b] (optional): 20 g (100 mL, 200 kcal)
- Total volume: 707 mL (807 mL with optional lipids)
- Total energy: 615 kcal (815 kcal with optional lipids)

(continued)

Box 4.6   Intradialytic Parenteral Nutrition (IDPN) Formulas: Examples for a 70-kg Patient (continued)

Low-Dextrose, Low-Calorie, and Low-Volume Formula
- Dextrose[a]: 45 g D_{70} (64 mL, 153 kcal)
- 1.3 g AA/kg: 90 g of 20% AA (450 mL, 360 kcal)
- 20% lipids[b] (optional): 12 g (60 mL, 120 kcal)
- Total volume: 514 mL (574 mL with optional lipids)
- Total energy: 513 kcal (633 kcal with optional lipids)

Abbreviations: AA: amino acids; D_{70}: 70% dextrose solution.
[a]The recommended amount of dextrose is 45–75 g per bag of IDPN.
[b]Lipids should provide <25% total calories.
Source: Reprinted with permission from reference 35: Byham–Gray L, Wiesen K, Stover J. *A Clinical Guide To Nutrition Care In Kidney Disease.* 2nd ed. Chicago, IL: Academy of Nutrition and Dietetics; 2013.

A more detailed discussion of IDPN administration is beyond the scope of this guide. Guidelines for administration and monitoring of IDPN (eg, formula calculations, infusion rates, metabolic and laboratory monitors) may be available from companies that provide IDPN (35).

Other Dialysis Schedules

Traditional home hemodialysis is comparable to thrice-weekly in-center hemodialysis (the most common schedule used in the United States). However, patients/clients may choose to dialyze more frequently, which may result in improved outcomes (40,41).

Short daily home hemodialysis may be performed five to six times per week for 2 to 3 hours per treatment (24,40,41).

Nocturnal hemodialysis (NHD) is currently performed two ways in the United States (35). In-center NHD is provided at a dialysis facility with a medical team (35). Nocturnal home hemodialysis (NHHD) is done in a patient's/client's home by the patient/client or the family (less than 2% of dialysis patients dialyze at home) (35). See Table 4.9 for a comparison of weekly HD treatment times between modalities (35,42,43). NHD, including NHHD, must be individualized for estimated dietary needs, ethnic/religious food preferences, and medical history (see Box 4.7 for guidelines) (35). As compared with thrice-weekly hemodialysis, the increased dialysis time of NHD may result in a decreased need for diet and fluid restrictions, but the individual's appetite may improve during NHD. This situation may make it difficult to control the patient's/client's dietary intake (35,42). Research on NHD suggests that more frequent dialysis, as provided in this modality, may result in improved clinical outcomes (35).

Table 4.9   Comparison of Hemodialysis Treatment Times

	Treatments/ Week	Treatment Duration, hours	Total Weekly Treatment Time, hours
Traditional HD	3	3–4	9–12
In-center NHD	3	8	24
NHHD	5–6	6–8	30–48

Abbreviations: HD, hemodialysis; NHD, nocturnal hemodialysis; NHHD, nocturnal home hemodialysis.
Source: Data are from references 35, 42, and 43.

Box 4.7   Guidelines for Nocturnal Hemodialysis Administered at Home

- Energy: 30–35 kcal/kg actual or adjusted body weight per day; adjust for weight loss/gain.
- Protein: 1.2 g protein per kilogram actual or adjusted body weight per day; adjust for additional protein needs.
- Fat: Lower serum triglycerides may be seen. If serum lipids are increased, intake of dietary fat and cholesterol should be limited.
- Fluid: Restriction is not necessary unless fluid intake exceeds maximum treatment fluid removal of 0.4 kg or 400 mL/h.
- Sodium: Amount is guided by fluid and blood pressure goals; normotensive patients/clients may need 1,500 to 2,300 mg/d.
- Potassium: Restriction is rarely needed but should be considered if hyperkalemia occurs; recommend augmented potassium intake in patients/clients with hypokalemia to limit problems such as muscle cramping.
- Phosphorus: Supplementation may be needed when dialyzing 5 or more nights a week.
- Vitamins: Renal multivitamin should be prescribed to replace water-soluble vitamins lost with dialysis.

Source: Data are from reference 35.

PLANNING THE NUTRITION PRESCRIPTION: KIDNEY TRANSPLANT

Boxes 4.8 and 4.9 (2,17,35,44) and the following sections review acute and chronic MNT recommendations for the patient/client after a kidney transplant.

**Box 4.8 Acute Phase[a] of Medical Nutrition Therapy After
Kidney Transplant**

Energy[b] (35,44)
- 1.3–1.5 × basal energy expenditure (BEE)
- 30–35 kcal/kg weight

Protein[b] (17,35,44)
- 1.3–2.0 g/kg weight with functioning allograft

Carbohydrate (44)
- 50%–70% of nonprotein calorics
- Carbohydrate-controlled diet as needed

Fat (44)
- 30%–50% of nonprotein calories

Fluid
- Ad lib (35,44)
- 1 mL/kg dry weight (44)
- Match output unless diuresis is goal (35,44)

Vitamins
- DRI (35)
- Supplementation is usually not necessary (44)
- ≥0.25 mcg vitamin D per day (17)

Minerals
- Sodium: ≤4 g/d (44); unrestricted if hypertension and edema are absent (35,44)
- Potassium: Unrestricted unless patient has hyperkalemia (44); if patient has hyperkalemia: <2.4 g/d (2)
- Calcium: 1,000–1,500 mg/d (35,44); supplement if necessary (44)
- Phosphorus: DRI (35); supplement if necessary (44)
- Magnesium: DRI (35); supplement if necessary (44)

---

[a]Acute phase = the eight weeks immediately posttransplant.
[b]Based on standard or adjusted body weight.
Source: Data are from references 2, 17, 35, and 44.

Box 4.9   Chronic Phase of Medical Nutrition Therapy After Kidney Transplant

Energy
- 23–35 kcal/kg/d (2)
- Achieve desirable body weight (35,44)
- Adjust for weight goals, age, gender, physical activity, and metabolic stressors (2)

Protein
- 0.8–1.0 g/kg/d with functioning allograft (2,35,44)

Carbohydrate
- 45%–50% of total calories (44)
- Promote whole grain intake (17)
- Fiber: 25 g/d for females; 30 g/d for males (17)

Fat
- Total fat: ≤30%–35% of total calories (17)
- PUFA: ≤8%–10% of total calories (17)
- MUFA: ≤20% of total calories (17)
- Saturated and *trans* fat: 8%–10% of total calories (17)
- Cholesterol: <300 mg/d (44)

Fluid
- Ad lib (44)

Vitamins
- DRI (35); supplement as needed (44)
- ≥ 0.25 mcg vitamin D per day (17)

Minerals
- Sodium: <2.4 g/d (2)
- Potassium: Supplement or restrict as needed (44); if patient has hyperkalemia: <2.4 g/d (2)
- Calcium: 2,000 mg/d
- Phosphorus: DRI (35); Replete with diet or a supplement as needed (2)
- Magnesium: DRI (35); Supplement or restrict as needed (44)

Source: Data are from references 2, 17, 35 and 44.

Protein Prescription

In the first 4 to 8 weeks after the transplant, the patient/ client should consume between 1.3 and 2.0 g protein per kg per day to reverse negative nitrogen balance and boost muscle mass (17,35,44). After surgical recovery, adult kidney transplant recipients with an adequately functioning transplanted kidney or allograft should consume 0.8 to 1.0 g protein per kg per day (2,35,44). Adequate, but not excessive, protein intake supports allograft survival and minimizes the risk of comorbid conditions (2).

Energy Prescription

It is important to use clinical judgment to determine the ideal edema-free body weight to use for energy calculations for patients/clients after a kidney transplant (2). Energy needs in the first 8 weeks after transplant are typically 30 to 35 kcal/kg/d (35,44). However, energy requirements during this time period may be higher when there are postoperative complications (35).

For the chronic posttransplant patient/client who has recovered from surgery, the RD should recommend between 23 and 35 kcal/kg/d (2). Maintenance of a desirable weight is an appropriate goal (35,44).

Carbohydrate Prescription

For posttransplant adults with diabetes, the RD should implement MNT for diabetes care to achieve a target A1c of approximately 7%. Intensive treatment of hyperglycemia while avoiding hypoglycemia prevents complications such as retinopathy and neuropathy, and it may slow the progression of established kidney disease. If the patient/ client develops new-onset diabetes after transplantation (NODAT), dietary carbohydrate should be prescribed as recommended for the care of diabetic patients/clients in general (2) and with the goal of preventing macrovascular complications (17).

Fat Prescription

Individuals with renal disease have a risk of heart disease equal to the risk for people with confirmed coronary heart disease (9). The fat prescription should set healthful targets for the amounts and types of fat consumed (ie, saturated, *trans*, polyunsaturated, and monounsaturated fat), with goal of improving lipid parameters (see Box 4.8) (17).

Evidence suggests that fish oil supplementation may be beneficial in reducing oxidative stress and improving lipid profile in adults after a kidney transplant (2).

Vitamin Prescription

Boxes 4.8 and 4.9 list vitamin recommendations for the patient/client who has had a kidney transplant.

- Sufficient vitamin D should be recommended to maintain levels of serum 25-hydroxyvitamin D equal to or greater than 30 ng/mL (2).
- Vitamin C supplementation is sometimes used to improve iron absorption for post–kidney transplant patients/clients who have iron-deficiency anemia (2). There is insufficient evidence to recommend vitamin C supplementation greater than the DRI in the management of iron-deficiency anemia, because supplemental vitamin C can increase the risk of hyperoxalosis (2).

When a posttransplant patient/client is assessed to be at higher nutritional risk due to poor dietary intake and decreasing GFR, the RD should recommend or prescribe a multivitamin preparation (2).

Electrolyte and Mineral Prescription

Boxes 4.8 and 4.9 list electrolyte and mineral recommendations for the patient/client who has had a kidney transplant.

Sodium

A sodium intake of less than 2.4 g/d is recommended for kidney transplant recipients after they recover from the acute phase. This target should be adjusted as appropriate based on fluid balance, blood pressure control, and other clinical findings (2). Some resources suggest dietary sodium intake can safely range from 2 to 4 g/d after a kidney transplant (35,44).

Potassium

A kidney transplant generally leads to normalized serum potassium levels, in which case dietary potassium restriction is not necessary (35). However, elevated serum potassium levels may be caused by a poorly functioning graft or adverse effects of medications such as calcineurin inhibitors (35). When a patient/client who has had a kidney transplant has hyperkalemia, the RD should recommend a potassium intake of less than 2.4g/d and consider other clinical factors, including serum potassium levels, medications that may affect potassium levels, glycemic control, and other issues (2).

Hypokalemia has also been reported in kidney transplant recipients and is likely caused by potassium-wasting diuretics (35). Hypokalemia or hyperkalemia can have direct effects on cardiac function, with a potential for cardiac arrhythmia and sudden death (2).

Calcium

After kidney transplant, calcium supplementation should be limited to 1,200-1,500 mg/d (35). For post–kidney transplant patients/clients, the RD should recommend a total elemental calcium intake (including dietary calcium, calcium supplementation, and calcium-based phosphate binders) of 2,000 mg/d or less (2,35,44). CKD patients/clients are predisposed to mineral and bone disorders. Serum calcium concentration is an important factor in regulating PTH secretion, which affects bone integrity and soft-tissue calcification (2). The RD should be aware of the risks of hypercalcemia, including soft-tissue calcification (2).

Phosphorus

Hypophosphatemia is most common in the early weeks after a kidney transplant (2). For adult kidney transplant recipients with low serum phosphorus, the RD should recommend/prescribe a high-phosphorus diet or supplements containing phosphorus (see Box 5.2 in Chapter 5) to replete serum phosphorus as needed (2). Generally, the DRI for phosphorus is appropriate for post–kidney transplant patients/clients (35).

Iron

Anemia guidelines from KDIGO in 2012 updated ferritin and TSAT cut-offs for patients/clients with CKD, but not for transplant patients specifically (33). According to the Academy's Evidence Analysis Library (EAL) CKD recommendations, when a posttransplant patient's/client's serum ferritin level is equal to or less than 100 ng/mL and his or her TSAT is equal to or less than 20%, oral or intravenous iron supplementation may be recommended (2).

The amount of iron supplementation recommended should maintain levels of serum iron that will adequately support erythropoiesis (2). Iron absorption may be impaired by other medications, such as phosphate binders (2).

Cardiovascular Disease Risk and the Post–Kidney Transplant Nutrition Prescription

The prevalence of both hypertension and hyperlipidemia (with risk for cardiovascular disease, coronary artery disease, and left ventricular hypertrophy) is higher in patients/clients with CKD, including post–kidney transplant patients/clients, compared with the general population. Dietary and other therapeutic lifestyle modifications are recommended as part of a comprehensive strategy to reduce cardiovascular disease risk in adults with CKD (9).

Enteral and Parenteral Nutrition Prescription

If enteral or parenteral nutrition is necessary after a kidney transplant, the nutrition prescription guidelines for the chronic posttransplant phase can be used (see Box 4.9).

CASE STUDY—NCP STEP 3, PART 1: PLANNING THE NUTRITION INTERVENTION

Full nutrition assessment data for this case study of a 56-year-old Cambodian woman with ESRD is presented at the end of Chapter 2. Nutrition diagnoses are listed at the end of Chapter 3.

Assessment Data Pertinent to the Nutrition Prescription

- Personal data: 56-year-old Cambodian woman.
- Anthropometric measurements: Height: 150 cm (59 inches); weight: 74.5 kg (admitting weight); EDW: 72 kg (stable); BMI: 32 (using EDW).

- Patient medical history: diabetes mellitus (DM), HTN, ESRD on PD, latent tuberculosis.
- Medications: Atorvastatin, renal MVI, $CaCO_3$, and Renagel (with meals); calcitriol; iron sulfate; NPH insulin with meals; isoniazid; vitamin B-6; lansoprazole.
- Current status: LEE (lower-extremity edema), facial edema, nausea/vomiting, febrile, peritonitis (third episode of peritonitis in 2 months).

Laboratory Values

Table 4.10 summarizes the patient's relevant laboratory test results.

Table 4.10   Laboratory Data Used in Nutrition Prescription for Case Study Patient

	Patient's Data (PD Reference Range)	Comments
Alb, g/dL	1.6 (≥3.5)	Consistent with peritonitis
Ca, mg/dL	8.8 (8.6–10.2)	Ca = 10.72 mg/dL when adjusted for low serum Alb[a]
PO_4, mg/dL	5.7 (3.5–5.5)	$Ca \times PO_4 = 61.1$ (goal <55)
K, mg/dL	4.2 (3.5–5)	K is normal; no restriction needed
Hgb, g/dL	9 (10–12)	Iron studies not available
Na, mmol/L	129 (134–143)	Consistent with bilateral LEE; facial edema

[a]Formula to adjust serum calcium for a low albumin value:
[(4 – Albumin) × 0.8] + Calcium = Adjusted Calcium.

Peritoneal Dialysis Regimen

Note: 2.5% dextrose provides 25 g dextrose per liter.
Sample calculation:

2 liters of 2.5% dextrose solution daily provides:

2 liters × (25 g dextrose per liter) = 50 g dextrose

(50 g dextrose per PD exchange) × (5 PD exchanges/d) =
250 g dextrose per day

(250 g dextrose per day) × (3.4 kcal per g dextrose) =
850 kcal/d

(850 kcal/d) × 70% absorption =
595 kcal/d from PD exchanges

Energy and Protein Needs

Using dry weight:

- Energy needs:

  ○ 72 kg × 25–30 kcal/kg/d = 1,800–2,160 kcal/d

  ○ Subtract 595 kcal provided by PD regime =
    1,205–1,565 kcal/d

- Protein needs:

  72 kg × 1.3 g/kg/d (due to peritonitis) = 94 g/d

Daily Peritoneal Dialysis Diet Prescription

Table 4.11 lists the patient's daily nutrient goals by food
group (45). Other elements of the daily prescription are
as follows:

- Based on the patient's past medical history and cal-
  culated macro- and micronutrient needs, suggest a
  renal, carbohydrate-controlled diabetic diet adjusted

to Cambodian food preferences as permissible within renal and diabetic requirements.

- Based on urine output of 500 mL/24 hours and edema/hyponatremia, suggest limiting dietary fluid intake to 1,000 mL/d.
- Based on edema/hyponatremia, suggest limiting dietary sodium to approximately 2 g/d.
- To prevent undesirable weight gain while maintaining dry weight, limit dietary calories to approximately 1,600 kcal/d. (Patient/client will receive an additional 595 kcal/d from PD exchanges.)
- To replete protein stores in the context of the diagnosis of peritonitis, provide approximately 94 g protein per day. Re-evaluate adequacy of estimated protein needs at nutrition follow-up.

Table 4.11 Case Study Diet Prescription by Nutrient and Food Group

	Servings	Protein, g	Energy, kcal	K, mg	PO₄, mg	Na, mg
Meat	10 oz	70	650	1,000	650	250
Milk[a]	4 oz	4	45	185	110	80
Fruit[b]	3	1.5	180	450–750	30	Trace
Vegetables[b]	3	3	75	450–750	60	45
Starch	8	16	640	280	280	640
Fat	1	0	45	10	5	55
Seasoning[c]	4	0	0	0	0	1,000
Totals:		**94.5 g**	**1,635 kcal**	**2,375–2,975 mg**	**1,135 mg**	**2,070 mg**

[a]Fat-free.
[b]Limit to one high-potassium fruit or vegetable per day (defined as ≥250 mg K per serving).
[c]Seasoning = salt.
Source: Data are from reference 45.

Chapter 5

Nutrition Intervention— Part Two: Implementation

This chapter offers suggestions for implementing nutrition interventions in each of the four domains of nutrition intervention for patients/clients with chronic kidney disease (CKD):

- Food and/or nutrient delivery
- Nutrition education
- Nutrition counseling
- Coordination of nutrition care

FOOD AND/OR NUTRIENT DELIVERY

Described as "an individualized approach for food/nutrient provision, including meals and snacks, enteral and parenteral feeding, and supplements," this domain of intervention can occur in many settings, including acute and chronic care, public health and other community settings, wellness programs, and policy development for all age groups (1). Categories in this domain that are frequently used in CKD include Supplements (ie, medical food supplements as well as vitamin and mineral supplements) and Nutrition-related medication management (eg, adjustment of phosphorus binders according to a physician-approved protocol, or recommendations for phosphorus supplements as appropriate for posttransplant patients/clients).

The intervention category of Enteral and parenteral nutrition may also be applied. Tables 4.4 and 4.5 in Chapter 4 summarize parenteral nutrition prescriptions that might be used in kidney disease. See Boxes 5.1 and 5.2 for information on oral supplement and enteral formula products (35). For the most current ingredient and nutrition analysis data for enteral nutrition products, consult manufacturers' Web sites.

Box 5.1   Oral Supplements and Enteral Formulas for Chronic Kidney Disease

Protein Modulars
- Example: Beneprotein[a]
- Characteristics: 100% high-quality whey protein.
- Indications: Inability to meet estimated protein requirements.

Energy, Other Modulars
- Example: Polycose[a]
  - Characteristics: Readily digestible carbohydrate.
  - Indications: Increased energy needs, inability to meet energy needs.
- Example: MCT oil[a]
  - Characteristics: Contains medium chain triglycerides (more readily hydrolyzed and absorbed).
  - Indications: Used when dietary fat is not well absorbed.

Oral Nutritional Supplements
- Examples: Milkshakes, Carnation Breakfast Essentials[a], Ensure[a], Nutren[a], Boost[a]
- Characteristics: Flavored for oral consumption. May contain milk. Most contain 1 kcal/mL and moderate protein levels.
- Indications: Inability to meet requirements via diet alone. Depending on level of kidney function and recommended use, micronutrient content should be evaluated closely.

(continued)

Box 5.1   Oral Supplements and Enteral Formulas for Chronic Kidney Disease (continued)

Standard Enteral Formulas
- Examples: Nutren 1.0[a], Osmolite[b], Isosource[a]
- Characteristics: 1 kcal/mL, moderate protein content. Most meet Dietary Reference Intakes for nutrients in <1,500 mL.
- Indications: Most patients requiring enteral feeding. Depending on level of kidney function and recommended use, micronutrient content should be evaluated closely.

Fluid-Restricted Formulas
- Examples: Nutren 2.0[a], TwoCal HN[b], Boost Plus[a]
- Characteristics: 1.5–2.0 kcal/mL, moderate protein content.
- Indications: Used in patients with fluid restriction. Depending on level of kidney function and recommended use, micronutrient content should be evaluated closely.

Fiber-Containing Supplements
- Examples: Jevity[b], Nutren with fiber[a]
- Characteristics: 1.0 kcal/mL, moderate protein. Type and amount of fiber may vary.
- Indications: May help normalize bowel function in some patients. Depending on level of kidney function and recommended use, micronutrient content should be evaluated closely.

Elemental and Peptide-Based
- Examples: Vivonex[a], Peptamen[a], Vital[b]
- Characteristics: 1.0 kcal/mL, moderate protein content. Protein source and type may vary.
- Indications: Used for patients with malabsorption and extreme GI dysfunction. Very unpalatable, but may be used orally in some patients.

Glucose Intolerance
- Example: Glucerna[b]
- Characteristics: Usually 1 kcal/mL but can vary; moderate protein content. Lower carbohydrate content than standard formulas.

(continued)

Box 5.1   Oral Supplements and Enteral Formulas for Chronic Kidney Disease (continued)

Glucose Intolerance (continued)
- Indications: May be effective in some enterally fed patients with difficult-to-control blood glucose. Depending on level of kidney function and recommended use, micronutrient content should be evaluated closely.

Specialized for CKD
- Examples: predialysis: Suplena[b], Renalcal[a]; on dialysis: Nepro[b]
- Characteristics: Protein and electrolytes modified. 1.8 to 2 kcal/mL.
- Indications: Useful in patients with difficult-to-control serum electrolyte levels.

Note: Manufacturers may change product formulations and offerings. Check product labels and Web sites for current information.
Manufacturers: [a]Nestle Nutrition, www.nestle-nutrition.com. [b]Abbott Nutrition, http://abbottnutrition.com.
Source: Data are from reference 35.

Box 5.2   Phosphorus Supplementation

Phos-NaK Powder[a]
- Product description: OTC; 1.5 g packets
- Electrolyte content per packet: Phosphorus: 8 mmol; potassium: 7.1 mEq; sodium: 164 mg
- Special instructions: Open packet and mix powder with 2.5 oz (75 mL) water or other liquid such as juice. Stir mixture well and drink.

K-Phos Original Dissolvable Tablets[b]
- Product description: Rx; tablets in 100- and 500-count bottles
- Electrolyte content per tablet: Phosphorus: 3.7 mmol; potassium: 3.7 mEq; sodium: 0 mg
- Special instructions: Add tablet to 6 to 8 oz (180 to 240 mL) water. Let tablets dissolve completely (this takes a few minutes), then stir and drink.

(continued)

Box 5.2   Phosphorus Supplementation (continued)

K-Phos MF[b]
- Product description: Rx; tablets in 100-count bottle
- Electrolyte content per tablet: Phosphorus: 4 mmol; potassium: 1.1 mEq; sodium: 67 mg

---

K-Phos No. 2[b]
- Product description: Rx; tablets in 100-count bottle
- Electrolyte content per tablet: Phosphorus: 8 mmol; potassium: 2.3 mEq; sodium: 134 mg

---

Phospha 250 Neutral[c]
- Product description: Rx; tablets in 100-count bottle
- Electrolyte content per tablet: Phosphorus: 8 mmol; potassium: 1.1 mEq; sodium: 298 mg

---

K-Phos Neutral[b]
- Product description: Rx; tablets in 100- and 500-count bottles
- Electrolyte content per tablet: Phosphorus: 8 mmol; potassium: 1.1 mEq; sodium: 298 mg

---

Abbreviations: OTC, over-the-counter; Rx, prescription.
Note: Manufacturers may change product formulations and offerings. Check product labels and Web sites for current information.
Manufacturers: [a]Cypress Pharmaceuticals, Madison, MS 39130; [b]Beach Pharmaceuticals, Tampa, FL 33681; Rising Pharmaceuticals, Allendale, NJ 07401.
Source: Data are from reference 35.

NUTRITION EDUCATION

The *IDNT Reference Manual* defines nutrition education as "a formal process to instruct or train a patient/client in a skill or to impart knowledge to help patients/clients voluntarily manage or modify food choices or eating behavior to maintain or improve health" (1). Suggested schedules for nutrition visits for medical nutrition therapy (MNT) in

CKD, which can be helpful in developing protocols for nutrition counseling and nutrition education, have been published (46). See Table 1.2 in Chapter 1 for information about the number of annual MNT visits that are approved for reimbursement under Medicare Part B guidelines.

Box 5.3 lists several major resources for nutrition education materials that target populations with CKD. The following brief discussions are intended to provide RDs with some suggested nutrition education topics and resources to support MNT recommendations from various evidence-based guidelines.

Box 5.3   **Nutrition Education Resources for Chronic Kidney Disease (CKD)[a]**

- **Academy of Nutrition and Dietetics**:
  - *Nutrition Care Manual.* Comprehensive online clinical nutrition manual with professional information and client handouts related to CKD. Subscription required. www.nutritioncaremanual.org.
  - *A Healthy Food Guide for People with Chronic Kidney Disease,* 2nd ed. (patient/client education booklet). www.eatright.org/shop.
  - *A Healthy Food Guide for People on Dialysis,* 2nd ed. (patient/client education booklet). www.eatright.org/shop.
- **American Academy of Kidney Patients (AAKP)**:
  A nonprofit. "The independent voice of kidney patients since 1969." *aakpRENALIFE* magazine available free online. Membership is free for patients/clients and family members. www.aakp.org/join.html.
- ***Journal of Renal Nutrition*, Collections, Patient Education Papers**: The journal is the professional publication of the National Kidney Foundation—Council on Renal Nutrition (NKF-CRN). Member log-in is not required for these papers. www.jrnjournal.org/content/patienteducation.

(continued)

Box 5.3   Nutrition Education Resources for Chronic Kidney Disease (CKD)[a] (continued)

- **Life Options**: A program of the Medical Education Institute (MEI). Includes links for Kidney School (interactive modules for patients/clients with CKD) and Home Dialysis Central (information about home dialysis in all modalities). www.lifeoptions.org.
- **MedLine Plus**: From US National Library of Medicine (NLM) and National Institutes of Health (NIH). www.nlm.nih.gov/medlineplus/kidneyfailure.html.
- **National Kidney Disease Education Program (NKDEP)**: From US Department of Health and Human Services (DHHS) and National Institute of Diabetes, Digestive and Kidney Diseases (NIDDK):
  ◦ Home page: www.nkdep.nih.gov/professionals/index.htm.
  ◦ Nutrition materials for professionals and patients/clients: www.nkdep.nih.gov/professionals/ckd-nutrition.htm.
- **National Kidney Foundation (NKF)**:
  ◦ Home page: www.kidney.org.
  ◦ Nutrition and diet information for patients/clients: www.kidney.org/atoz/atozTopic_Nutrition-Diet.cfm.
- **Renal Practice Group (RPG), Academy of Nutrition and Dietetics**: Patient/client education materials available to RPG members only. www.renalnutrition.org.
- **Web sites of dialysis providers**: Many of their materials are proprietary and subject to change. RDs are encouraged to check for materials as needed.

[a]This list is not meant to be all-inclusive. It identifies major sources of materials that are useful in nutrition education and counseling related to CKD or end-stage renal disease.

Weight Management

Weight Loss

Weight loss therapy, when appropriate, should be individualized. Discussions of label reading, alternative approaches to weight loss, and physical activity goals can be useful. For more information on physical activity, see Table 5.1 and Box 5.4 (23). Interventions to consider when PD patients/clients need to lose weight include the following (47):

- Increase activity as approved by the physician.
- Limit sodium and fluid to reduce the need for higher-percentage dextrose exchanges.
- Consider alternate osmotic agents such as icodextrin.
- Control energy intake to support weight loss.
- Reduce intake of sugars, fats, and foods of low nutrient density.

Table 5.1　Physical Activity (PA) Intervention Strategies for Weight Control in Adults

Goal	Physical Activity Strategy
Prevention of weight gain	• 150–250 min PA per week (1,200–1,500 kcal/wk) prevents weight gain greater than 3% in most adults.
Weight loss	• PA <150 min/wk promotes minimal weight loss. • PA >150 min/wk results in modest weight loss (~2–3 kg). • PA >225–420 min/wk results in 5–7.5 kg weight loss, and a dose response exists.
Weight maintenance after weight loss	• During weight maintenance, a minimum of approximately 200–300 minutes PA per week may reduce weight regain after weight loss; however, more PA is better.

Source: Reprinted with permission from reference 23: Franz MJ, Boucher JL, Pereira RF. *ADA Pocket Guide to Lipid Disorders, Hypertension, Diabetes, and Weight Management.* Chicago, IL: American Dietetic Association; 2011:26.

Box 5.4　Physical Activity Guidelines

Adults
- Engage in 2½ hours of moderate-intensity aerobic physical activity[a] or 1¼ hours of vigorous-intensity physical activity[b] per week.

(continued)

Box 5.4 Physical Activity Guidelines (continued)

Adults (continued)
- Aerobic activity should be performed in episodes at least 10 minutes in duration.
- For more extensive health benefits, increase aerobic physical activity to 5 hours of moderate-intensity or 2½ hours of vigorous-intensity physical activity per week.
- Incorporate muscle-strengthening activities[c] at least 2 days per week.

Older Adults
- When physically capable, follow the guidelines for other adults.
- If older adults have a chronic condition that prohibits their ability to follow guidelines, they should be as physically active as abilities and conditions allow.
- If older adults are at risk of falling, they should do exercises to maintain and improve balance.

Adults with Disabilities
- If able, do 2½ hours of moderate-intensity aerobic activity[a] or 1¼ hours of vigorous-intensity activity[b] per week.
- Incorporate muscle-strengthening activities[c] involving all major groups at least 2 days per week.
- If adults are not able to meet these guidelines, they should engage in regular physical activity according to their abilities and avoid inactivity.

People with Chronic Medical Conditions
- Seek the important health benefits of regular physical activity under the guidance of a health care provider.

[a]Moderate-intensity activities for adults include walking briskly, water aerobics, ballroom dancing, and general gardening.
[b]Vigorous-intensity activities for adults include race walking, jogging or running, swimming laps, jumping rope, or hiking uphill or with a heavy backpack.
[c]Muscle-strengthening activities for adults include weight training, push-ups, sit-ups, and carrying heavy loads or heavy gardening.
Source: Adapted with permission from reference 23: Franz MJ, Boucher JL, Pereira RF. *ADA Pocket Guide to Lipid Disorders, Hypertension, Diabetes, and Weight Management.* Chicago, IL: American Dietetic Association; 2011:25–26.

Weight Gain

When patients/clients are underweight, RDs can work with them to identify means to improve energy intake. Appetite stimulants may also be appropriate, although it is important to understand their potential adverse effects (see Box 5.5) (35).

Box 5.5   Appetite Stimulants and Their Adverse Effects

---

megestrol acetate (Megace)
- Constipation, diarrhea, dyspepsia, hyperglycemia, nausea and vomiting.
- Blood clots in sedentary individuals.

---

dronabinol (Marinol)
- Seizure and seizure-like activity.
- Abdominal pain, dizziness, euphoria, somnolence, paranoia, tachycardia, and central nervous system effects (amnesia, changes in mood, confusion, delusions, hallucinations, mental depression, nervousness, or anxiety).
- Sleep disturbances may occur after discontinuation of therapy.

---

mirtazapine (Remeron)
- Abnormal dreams and/or thinking, dizziness, drowsiness, constipation, flu-like symptoms, dry mouth, increased appetite, and weight gain.
- **Note**: This drug is an antidepressant that may be used for appetite stimulation because of its side effects of increased appetite and weight gain.

Source: Adapted with permission from reference 35: Byham-Gray L, Wiesen K, Stover J. *A Clinical Guide To Nutrition Care In Kidney Disease.* 2nd ed. Chicago, IL: Academy of Nutrition and Dietetics; 2013.

Protein, Fat, Carbohydrate, and Fiber Intake

Exchange lists such as those in *A Healthy Food Guide for People with CKD* and *A Healthy Food Guide for People on Dialysis* can be useful in patient/client education (see Box 5.3 and Table 5.2) (47).

Table 5.2   National Renal Diet Exchanges for Chronic Kidney Disease (CKD)[a]

Food Group	Protein, g	Calories	Na, mg	K, mg	PO_4, mg
Protein	6–8	50–100	20–150	50–150	50–100
High-PO_4 protein	6–8	50–100	20–150	50–350	100–300
High-Na protein	6–8	50–100	200–450	50–150	50–100
Vegetarian protein	6–8	70–150	10–200	60–150	80–150
High-Na/K/PO_4	6–8	70–150	250–400	250–500	200–400
Vegetables:					
low K	2–3	10–100	0–50	20–150	10–70
medium K	2–3	10–100	0–50	150–250	10–70
high K	2–3	10–100	0–50	250–550	10–70
Fruit:					
low K	0–1	20–100	0–10	20–150	1–20
medium K	0–1	20–100	0–10	150–250	1–20
high K	0–1	20–100	0–10	250–550	1–20
Breads and starches	2–3	50–200	0–150	10–100	10–70
High Na, PO_4	2–3	50–200	150–400	10–100	100–200
Calorie boosters	0–1	100–150	0–100	0–100	0–100
Flavor	0	0–20	250–300	0–100	0–20

[a]Nutrient information is per serving.

Source: Adapted with permission from reference 45: American Dietetic Association. *National Renal Diet: Professional Guide*. 2nd ed. Chicago, IL: American Dietetic Association; 2002.

Table 4.6 in Chapter 4 summarizes MNT priorities for hemodialysis (HD) and peritoneal dialysis (PD), including goals for dietary fat. Education materials from the National Cholesterol Education Program (NCEP) can be applied in CKD, with modification as needed for the special needs of this population (see Box 5.3 and the reference list).

Carbohydrate intake may be addressed as part of nutrition education for CKD patients/clients with diabetes. Box 5.6 presents some guidelines for integrating CKD and diabetes education, as adapted from KDOQI's diabetes guidelines (4).

**Box 5.6   Components and Principles of Diabetes and Chronic
            Kidney Disease (CKD) Self-Management**

- Describe the disease processes for diabetes and CKD, as well as treatment options.
- Provide explanations in lay terminology and evaluate the patient's understanding. Assess and address beliefs about the nature, cause, and treatment of the illness. Explain consequences of nonadherence.
- Promote social support by involving significant others in educational activities.
- Incorporate appropriate nutritional management. Attention should be paid to cultural food preferences in nutrition counseling.
- Describe purpose and side effects of medicines. Include caregivers. Explain that health care providers and the patient work together to find the right treatment regimen.
- Discuss importance of self-monitoring of glucose. Describe symptoms of hyper- and hypoglycemia. Assess patient awareness of hypoglycemia.
- Review prevention, detection, and treatment of further diabetes complications.
- Encourage risk reduction behavior, such as smoking cessation, exercise, weight loss, and continued management of nutrition and medications.

(continued)

**Box 5.6   Components and Principles of Diabetes and Chronic
Kidney Disease (CKD) Self-Management** (continued)

- Support problem solving and goal setting. Establish a step-wise approach to easily achievable goals. Encourage discussion of barriers (such as transportation, financial issues, social support) and refer as appropriate.
- Integrate psychosocial evaluation and refer as appropriate.
- Promote preconception care, management during pregnancy, and gestational diabetes management as appropriate.

Source: Reprinted from Table 56 in reference 5: National Kidney Foundation. KDOQI clinical practice guidelines and clinical practice recommendations for diabetes and chronic kidney disease. *Am J Kidney Dis.* 2007;49(2 suppl 2):S1–S180. www.kidney.org/professionals/kdoqi/guideline_diabetes/cpr4 .htm#tab56. Reprinted with permission from National Kidney Foundation, Inc.

Due to restrictions on dietary phosphorus intake, many CKD patients/clients have difficulty achieving adequate dietary fiber. Helpful nutrition education tools are available on the Web pages of some dialysis providers or in other Internet sites as noted in Box 5.3.

Sodium, Potassium, Phosphorus, and Other Minerals

Recommendations for sodium, potassium, phosphorus, and other minerals for different stages of the CKD spectrum and for different modalities of renal replacement therapy (RRT) are summarized in Chapter 4. Exchange lists for renal diets can be used to teach patients/clients how to select foods when sodium, potassium, and phosphorus must be controlled (see Table 5.2). RDs can make further adjustments to address individual economic, cultural, and other considerations.

Nutrition education for phosphorus control in CKD stage 5 can inform patients/clients about food sources of phosphorus and enable them to adjust phosphorus-binder doses according to intake (see Box 2.2 in Chapter 2 for basic information about binders).

Calcium

RDs can provide practical advice to CKD patients/clients about how to achieve recommended goals for calcium intake of less than 2,000 mg/d (2,10). The RD should educate patients/clients about calcium from all sources, including diet and medications such as phosphorus binders (see Box 2.2 in Chapter 2).

Iron

Patients/clients may be instructed to take iron supplements to maintain adequate serum iron levels. See Table 5.3 for more information on common iron supplements (24).

Table 5.3   Common Oral Iron Supplements

Selected Products (Iron Compound)	% Elemental Iron
Ferro-Sequels[a], Hemocyte, Nephro-Fer (ferrous fumarate)	33%
FE-40, Fergon (ferrous gluconate)	12%
Feosol, tablet or capsule; Slow Fe (ferrous sulfate)	20%
Proferrin (heme iron polypeptide)	N/A (12 mg elemental iron per tablet)
EzFe, Ferrex 150, Niferex, Niferex-150 (iron polysaccharide complex)	Iron is 100% elemental

N/A, not available.
[a]Contains docusate.
Source: Data are from reference 24.

Vitamins

As mentioned in Chapter 4, the Evidenced-Based Nutrition Practice Guidelines (EBNPG) for CKD provide detailed recommendations for vitamin B intake as well as vitamin C. See the Appendix of this guide for information about some common preparations of renal-specific multivitamins. Supplementation for vitamin C should not exceed 60 mg per day (31). The RD can inform patients/clients about standards to assess vitamin D nutrition in CKD and about recommended repletion of vitamin D in accordance with the EBNPG for CKD (10,16).

Medications and Food Safety After Kidney Transplant

Immunosuppressants for individuals who have had a kidney transplant have numerous adverse effects that will respond to nutrition interventions (see Box 5.7) (4). Transplant patients/clients are at increased risk of foodborne illness and should be carefully educated about basic food safety (see Box 5.8) (44,48).

Box 5.7   Potential Nutrition-Related Adverse Effects of Immunosuppressants and Possible Interventions

Cyclosporin A (Sandimmune, Neoral[a])
- Hyperkalemia: Restrict potassium intake.
- Hyperglycemia: Monitor blood glucose levels. Address carbohydrate load and distribution.
- Gingival hyperplasia: Encourage good oral hygiene.
- Hypertension: Restrict sodium intake.
- Hypomagnesemia: Suggest magnesium supplements.
- Gastrointestinal distress: Provide nutrient-dense foods that patient/client will eat. Ensure adequate protein and fluid intake.
- Hyperlipidemia: Suggest therapeutic lifestyle changes.

(continued)

**Box 5.7   Potential Nutrition-Related Adverse Effects of
             Immunosuppressants and Possible Interventions**
             (continued)

Azathioprine (Imuran[b])
- Infection: Provide nutrient-dense foods that patient/client will eat.
- Mouth ulcers: Modify diet texture.
- Folate deficiency: Suggest folate supplements.
- Gastrointestinal distress: Provide nutrient-dense foods that patient/client will eat. Ensure adequate protein and fluid intake.

Corticosteroids (Prednisone[c], Prednisolone[c], Solu-Medrol[d])
- Cushingoid appearance: Address carbohydrate load and increase protein intake.
- Sodium retention: Restrict sodium intake.
- Enhanced appetite: Suggest low-calorie snacks and eating behavior modification.
- Hyperlipidemia: Limit fat intake to <30% calories during long-term phase.
- Hyperglycemia: Monitor blood glucose levels. Address carbohydrate load and distribution.
- Protein catabolism: Increase protein provision.
- Gastrointestinal ulceration: Limit/restrict caffeine if patient has caffeine sensitivity.
- Bone loss: Ensure adequate calcium and vitamin D intake; consider need for bisphosphonates, calcitriol, and estrogen or testosterone.

Tacrolimus (Prograf, FK506[e])
- Hypertension: Restrict sodium intake.
- Hyperglycemia: Monitor blood glucose levels and address carbohydrate load and distribution.
- Hyperlipidemia: Limit fat intake to <30% calories during long-term phase.
- Hyperkalemia: Restrict potassium intake.
- Hypomagnesemia: Suggest magnesium supplements.
- Gastrointestinal distress: Provide nutrient-dense foods that patient/client will eat. Ensure adequate protein and fluid intake.

(continued)

**Box 5.7   Potential Nutrition-Related Adverse Effects of
Immunosuppressants and Possible Interventions**
(continued)

**Mycophenolate mofetil (Cellcept, RS-61443[f]);
antithymocyte Globulin (ATG[g]); muromonab-CD3
(Orthoclone OKT3[h]); daclizumab (Zenepax[f]); basiliximab
(Simulect[a])**

- Gastrointestinal distress: Provide nutrient-dense foods that
  patient/client will eat. Ensure adequate protein and fluid
  intake.

Sirolimus (Rapamune[i])

- Hyperlipidemia: Monitor blood glucose levels. Address carbohydrate load and distribution.
- Delayed wound healing: Suggest vitamin supplementation
  and increased protein intake.
- Hypokalemia: Suggest potassium supplements.

Manufacturers: [a]Novartis Pharmaceuticals, East Hanover, NJ 07936; [b]Bedford Laboratories, Bedford, OH 44146; [c]Rixabe Laboratories, Columbus, OH 43228; [d]Pfizer, New York, NY 10017; [e]Astellas Pharma US, Deerfield, IL 60015; [f]Novartis Pharmaceuticals, East Hanover, NJ; [g]Upjohn, Kalamazoo, MI 49001; [h]Ortho Biotech, Bridgewater, NJ 08807-0914; [i]Wyeth Pharmaceuticals, Philadelphia, PA 19101.
Source: Data are from reference 35.

**Box 5.8   Food Safety Recommendations for
Immunosuppressed Individuals**

Avoid the following:
- All raw and undercooked meats (especially ground or
  chopped), poultry, fish, and game
- Sushi, raw seafood, and shellfish
- Raw or undercooked eggs and foods containing them (such
  as home-made eggnog, caesar dressing)
- All unpasteurized milk and dairy products
- Unpasteurized juices and ciders
- All fresh, uncooked sprouts (bean, alfalfa, others)

(continued)

**Box 5.8   Food Safety Recommendations for
            Immunosuppressed Individuals** (continued)

Avoid the following: (continued)
- Raw or spoiled food items
- Food contaminated with a foodborne illness
- Outdated packaged foods
- Food from dented or otherwise damaged containers

Always practice the following:
- Use safe food-handling methods (see www.foodsafety.gov)
- Store food promptly and appropriately
- Use leftovers within 1 to 2 days
- Avoid buffet-style meals, salad bars, potlucks
- Drink water from safe sources

Source: Data are from reference 44.

NUTRITION COUNSELING

In the Nutrition Counseling domain, the RD's intervention moves beyond strengthening the patient's/client's knowledge base to helping the patient/client set priorities and develop behaviors that support on-going care. In the *IDNT Reference Manual,* nutrition counseling is described as "a supportive process, characterized by a collaborative counselor-patient relationship to establish food, nutrition and physical activity priorities, goals, and individualized action plans that acknowledge and foster responsibility for self-care to treat an existing condition and promote health" (1).

The following material from *ADA Pocket Guide to Lipid Disorders, Hypertension, Diabetes, and Weight Management* (23) summarizes an organized approach to evaluate patient/client readiness for counseling and to determine behavior change strategies. The following

"5 A's" describe steps that can guide the RD in starting an education/counseling session and implementing the best of several behavioral change strategies for each part of the session (49).

- Step 1: Ask
- Step 2: Assess
- Step 3: Advise
- Step 4: Agree
- Step 5: Arrange

Taken together, these 5 A's provide a workable framework that can integrate other counseling models.

Step 1: Ask

The "ask" step emphasizes the importance of asking questions as the RD aims to develop a relationship with the patient/client. The following tactics are essential to this step:

- Use motivational interview techniques (Box 5.9) (23) throughout the nutrition education/counseling session (50,51).
- Establish rapport by demonstrating the ability to be open, genuine, caring, and empathetic.
- Begin each session by asking questions to determine what the patient/client wants to know and accomplish and what you can do to be of assistance.

Box 5.9   Motivational Interviewing Techniques

Ask Open-Ended Questions
- Encourage patients/clients to do the talking.
- Do not ask questions that elicit a "yes" or "no" response.

(continued)

Box 5.9 Motivational Interviewing Techniques (continued)

Express Empathy
- Acknowledge the patient's/client's difficulties.
- Validate the patient's/client's thoughts and feelings.

Listen Reflectively
- Rephrase the patient's/client's responses to reflect what you think you heard.
- State back what you think the patient/client meant.

Support Self-Efficacy
- Provide choices and reassure the patient/client about expected outcomes.

Express Sympathy
- Express acceptance and understanding.
- Use reflective listening and expect ambivalence.

Explore Discrepancies
- Let individuals explore their reasons for changing or not changing behaviors.

Roll with Resistance
- Avoid arguments.
- Avoid judging and labeling.
- Change strategies if individuals show resistance.

Summarize
- Rephrase the overall content and meaning of the conversation.
- Reveal any ambiguity.

Promote Empowerment
- Recognize that individuals are the source of their own solutions, and each individual is in charge of and responsible for his or her own care.

Source: Adapted with permission from reference 23: Franz MJ, Boucher JL, Pereira RF. *ADA Pocket Guide to Lipid Disorders, Hypertension, Diabetes, and Weight Management.* Chicago, IL: American Dietetic Association; 2011.

Step 2: Assess

In the "assess" step, the RD evaluates the patient's/client's readiness to change (Box 5.10) (52,53) as part of the nutrition assessment (see Chapter 2 for more information on nutrition assessment).

Box 5.10   Transtheoretical Model of Intentional Behavior Change (Stages of Change)

Precontemplation
- Attitude toward lifestyle change is "Never": Patient/client has no intention of changing behavior in foreseeable future. He or she is unaware of problem or resistant to efforts to modify behavior.
- Interventions for health professionals:
  ○ Personalize risk factors.
  ○ Discuss health concern(s) and implications.

Contemplation
- Attitude toward lifestyle change is "Someday": Patient/client is aware there is a problem and is seriously thinking about change, but has no commitment to action in near future.
- Interventions for health professionals:
  ○ Provide basic information.
  ○ Demonstrate that the pros of change outweigh the cons.

Preparation
- Attitude toward lifestyle change is "Soon": Patient/client is prepared to make decisions and is committed to action in the next 30 days; he or she begins small behavioral changes.
- Interventions for health professionals:
  ○ Establish a start date.
  ○ Teach specific "how-to" skills.

(continued)

Box 5.10   **Transtheoretical Model of Intentional Behavior Change (Stages of Change)** (continued)

Action
- Attitude toward lifestyle change is "Now": Patient/client demonstrates notable overt efforts to change and targets behaviors that can be modified to acceptable criteria. He or she may not consistently carry out new behaviors.
- Interventions for health professionals:
  - Implement counseling strategies.
  - Continue to reinforce and support decision to change.
  - Discuss difference between a lapse and a relapse.

Maintenance
- Attitude toward lifestyle change is "Forever": Patient/client is working to stabilize behavior change and avoid relapse and maintains behavior change for at least 6 months.
- Interventions for health professionals:
  - Provide support; encourage behavior maintenance strategies.
  - Continue relapse prevention counseling.

Source: Adapted with permission from reference 23: Franz MJ, Boucher JL, Pereira RF. *ADA Pocket Guide to Lipid Disorders, Hypertension, Diabetes, and Weight Management.* Chicago, IL: American Dietetic Association; 2011.

When using Stages of Change, the RD's objective is to help the patient/client achieve the action or maintenance stage for the desired behavior:

- If patients/clients are in the **precontemplation** stage, the goal is to help them recognize they are at risk for a health problem.
- If patients/clients are in the **contemplation** stage, aim to help them believe their risk of disease is serious and that personal actions make a difference.

The benefits must outweigh the barriers to patients/clients before they will take the next step.

- If patients/clients are in the **preparation** stage, provide encouragement and set a start date.
- If patients/clients are in the **action** stage, help them implement the strategies that individuals who have made lifestyle changes identify as the most helpful (Box 5.11) (54,55). Use tools such as the following:
  - Food and activity records so the patient/client becomes aware of changes he or she needs and is willing to make (also helpful in the preparation stage)
  - Goal setting so the patient/client determines to make realistic changes
- If patients/clients are in the **maintenance** stage, provide support and continue encouragement to facilitate behaviors that maintain the healthful change (Box 5.12) (54,55).

Box 5.11   Strategies for Modifying Behavior

Self-Monitoring
- Record target behaviors and associated factors to increase awareness of behavior; participants report this strategy to be helpful.
- Record the "what, where, and when" of eating and physical activity (individuals with diabetes should also keep blood glucose monitoring records).

Goal Setting
- Set specific short-term targets for behavior habits to achieve incremental improvements.

(continued)

Box 5.11   Strategies for Modifying Behavior (continued)

Stimulus Control
- Identify triggers for problem behaviors; design strategies to break links.
- Restrict environmental factors associated with inappropriate behaviors.
- Eat at specific times; set aside time and place for physical activities.
- Avoid purchasing foods that are perceived as difficult to eat in moderation.

Cognitive Restructuring
- Change perceptions, thoughts, or beliefs that undermine your behavior-change efforts.
- Change thinking patterns from unrealistic goals to realistic and achievable goals.
- Move thinking patterns away from self-rejection and toward self-acceptance.

Contingency Management
- Use rewards (tangible or verbal) to improve performance of specific behaviors or recognize when specified goals are reached (participants rated this strategy as least helpful).
- Create contracts to formalize agreements; contracts should be short-term and focus on increasing healthful behaviors.

Stress Management
- Stress is a primary predictor of relapse; therefore, methods to reduce stress and tension are critical.
- Try tension reduction skills such as diaphragmatic breathing, progressive muscle relaxation, and/or meditation.
- Regular physical activity helps reduce stress.

Source: Adapted with permission from reference 23: Franz MJ, Boucher JL, Pereira RF. *ADA Pocket Guide to Lipid Disorders, Hypertension, Diabetes, and Weight Management.* Chicago, IL: American Dietetic Association; 2011.

Box 5.12   Strategies for Maintaining Behavior Change

Structured Programs with Ongoing Contact
- Individuals aiming to achieve and maintain goals require assistance from structured programs with consistent follow-up contacts.
- Maintain visits, telephone calls, or Internet communication to promote adherence with recommended lifestyle changes.

Social Support
- Use social support—family, peer support, self-help or work-site groups, or involvement in social activities—to maintain successful behavior change.

Physical Activity and Exercise
- Promote regular involvement in physical activities—individuals who exercise regularly are also more likely to maintain other health behaviors.

Relapse Prevention
- Recognize that lapses in behavior can be anticipated in certain situations (eg, travel, social situations, celebrations, stressful situations, loneliness) and develop skills for those situations.
- Individuals can practice coping strategies to handle high-risk situations (eg, stress management, social situation skills).

Source: Adapted with permission from reference 23: Franz MJ, Boucher JL, Pereira RF. *ADA Pocket Guide to Lipid Disorders, Hypertension, Diabetes, and Weight Management.* Chicago, IL: American Dietetic Association; 2011.

Step 3: Advise

The "advise" step uses a client-centered framework:

- Focus on the concerns of the patient/client.
- Allow the patient/client to be the expert for him- or herself.

- Adapt nutrition interventions to meet the patient's/client's needs, wants, priorities, preferences, and expectations.

Step 4: Agree

In the "agree" step, the RD facilitates the patient's/client's process of setting his or her own short-term goals related to nutrition, physical activity, or monitoring of pertinent laboratory tests (as appropriate), and helps outline the patient's/client's potential methods for accomplishing a lifestyle change. Scaling questions are recommended. For example:

- "On a scale of zero to 10, with zero being not important and 10 being very important, how important is it for you to modify XX behavior?" can be used to evaluate a patient's/client's goals.
- "On a scale of zero to 10, with zero being not important and 10 being very important, how confident are you that you can XX?" can be used to evaluate a patient's/client's plans.

Step 5: Arrange

In the "arrange" step, the RD helps implement a plan for follow-up adapted to the patient's/client's goals and needs, the patient's/client's level of support from family and friends, and the available resources. Crucial tasks include the following:

- Schedule follow-up visits.
- Provide contact information for future questions.
- Make referrals and/or provide contact information for other providers.

COORDINATION OF NUTRITION CARE

The fourth and final domain of nutrition intervention is defined as "consultation with, referral to, or coordination of nutrition care with other health care providers, institutions, or agencies that can assist in treating or managing nutrition-related problems" (1). Given the long-term relationship between RDs in dialysis centers and their patients/clients, there can be many intervention opportunities over the years in this domain. Professional partners in coordinated care may include staff at home health agencies and long-term care facilities, other health care professionals specializing in diabetes care, other RDs working in community settings such as Meals on Wheels, or RDs in other specialties such as weight management, liver disease, or other areas.

CASE STUDY—NCP STEP 3, PART 2: IMPLEMENTING THE NUTRITION INTERVENTION

Full assessment data for this case study of a 56-year-old Cambodian woman with ESRD is presented at the end of Chapter 2; nutrition diagnoses are listed at the end of Chapter 3; and the nutrition intervention plan is described at the end of Chapter 4. This note addresses the domains of Nutrition Education and Nutrition Counseling. Although Coordination of Care is not an intervention at this time, it may be addressed in future documentation.

Nutrition Education Intervention

- Explain to the patient the nutrition prescription modifications needed to reduce dietary phosphorus.
- Explain to the patient how her protein needs have increased because of peritonitis, and also educate her

about the need to keep her phosphorus intake as low as possible.

- Help the patient identify methods to control nausea symptoms, such as switching to a non-cola carbonated beverage to reduce phosphorus intake and eating a moderate amount of low-sodium crackers.
- Explain findings from routine laboratory tests and teach the patient how she can adjust her diet in accordance with laboratory results.

Nutrition Counseling Intervention

- Use Motivational Interviewing to determine how well the patient has accepted her diagnosis and her ability to recognize the changes needed in her diet.
- Use Motivational Interviewing to assure the patient that she can exercise her freedom of choice about how to use information that is provided regarding outcomes (eg, laboratory values) and diet.

Chapter 6

Nutrition Monitoring and Evaluation

Nutrition monitoring and evaluation determine whether a patient/client is meeting the agreed-upon nutrition goals or outcomes. In chronic kidney disease (CKD), a patient's/client's progress toward specific reference standards must be determined as part of monitoring and evaluation (1).

Outcomes and acceptable goals may change as a patient/client moves from one stage of CKD to the next or as treatment modalities change (eg, medical management, hemodialysis [HD], peritoneal dialysis [PD], or transplantation). Following is a list of potential outcomes that may be used for monitoring the patient/client with CKD (1):

- Food and nutrition-related history: Changes in energy, fluid, macronutrient, and micronutrient intake; Food and nutrition knowledge, beliefs, and attitudes; Estimated energy, macronutrient, fluid and micronutrient needs
- Changes in biochemical data, medical tests, and procedures
- Changes in anthropometric measurements
- Nutrition-focused physical findings

When accepted evidence-based standards are used, monitoring and evaluation of the aforementioned factors can determine the effectiveness of medical nutrition therapy (MNT) in adults who have CKD and those who are post–kidney transplant.

MONITORING AND EVALUATION RECOMMENDATIONS

Specific nutrition monitoring and evaluation recommendations for patients/clients with CKD can be found in the Evidence-Based Nutrition Practice Guidelines (EBNPG) for CKD and the NKF-KDOQI nutrition guidelines (2,3). See Box 6.1 for recommendations from the EBNPG (2). The NKF-KDOQI nutrition guidelines suggest monitoring several parameters for CKD and dialysis patients/clients (3). For nutrition monitoring and evaluation, the registered dietitian (RD) should follow up with individuals with CKD at regular intervals. Box 2.7 in Chapter 2 lists biochemical parameters that may be monitored in CKD, with suggestions about why each parameter is utilized. Box 6.2 suggests how often certain parameters may be evaluated in CKD (3).

Box 6.1   Nutrition Monitoring and Evaluation Recommendations from the Evidence-Based Nutrition Practice Guidelines for Chronic Kidney Disease

The registered dietitian (RD) should monitor and evaluate various biochemical parameters in adults with chronic kidney disease (CKD), including post–kidney transplant, related to:
- Glycemic control
- Protein-energy malnutrition
- Inflammation
- Kidney function
- Mineral and bone disorders
- Anemia

(continued)

Box 6.1   Nutrition Monitoring and Evaluation
Recommendations from the Evidence-Based Nutrition
Practice Guidelines for Chronic Kidney Disease
(continued)

- Dyslipidemia
- Electrolyte disorders
- Others as appropriate

The RD should monitor the following in adults with CKD, including post–kidney transplant:
- Food and nutrient intake (eg, diet history, diet experience, and intake of calcium, phosphorus and others, as appropriate) and intake of macronutrients and micronutrients, such as energy, protein, sodium, potassium
- Medication (prescription and over-the-counter), dietary supplement (vitamin, minerals, protein, etc), and herbal or botanical supplement use
- Knowledge, beliefs, or attitudes (eg, readiness to change nutrition and lifestyle behaviors)
- Behavior
- Factors affecting access to food and food- and nutrition-related supplies (eg, safe food and meal availability).

Source: Data are from reference 2.

Box 6.2   Recommended Measures for Monitoring Nutritional
Status of Maintenance Dialysis Patients/Clients[a]

Category 1. Routine Measurements[b]
- Predialysis or stabilized serum albumin: Measure at least once a month.
- % of usual post–hemodialysis (HD) or post–peritoneal dialysis (PD) drain body weight: Measure at least once a month.
- Subjective global assessment (SGA): Measure at least every 4 months.
- Dietary interview and/or diary: Measure at least every 6 months.
- Normalized protein nitrogen appearance (nPNA): Measure at least every 6 months.

(continued)

Box 6.2   **Recommended Measures for Monitoring Nutritional Status of Maintenance Dialysis Patients/Clients**[a] (continued)

---

2. Measures to Confirm or Extend the Data from the Category 1 Measurements
- Predialysis or stabilized serum prealbumin: Measure at least monthly in HD; at least every 3–4 months in PD.
- Skinfold thickness: Measure as needed.
- Mid-arm muscle area, circumference, or diameter: Measure as needed.
- Dual energy X-ray absorptiometry: Measure as needed.

---

3. Other Clinically Useful Measures
Note: Low values in this category might suggest the need for more rigorous examination of protein-energy nutritional status. Measure as needed.

- Predialysis or stabilized serum creatinine
- Predialysis or stabilized serum urea nitrogen
- Predialysis or stabilized serum cholesterol
- Creatinine index

---

[a]The Centers for Medicare & Medicaid Services have established a Measures Assessment Tool (MAT), which outlines specific time frames for nutrition monitoring for dialysis patients/clients (www.cms.gov/Medicare/Provider-Enrollment-and-Certification/GuidanceforLawsAndRegulations/Dialysis.html). According to MAT, the following should be monitored monthly: albumin, body weight, calcium, and phosphorus. Hemoglobin should be monitored monthly in patients who are not on erythropoiesis-stimulating agent (ESA) and those on ESA who are stable. Monitor hemoglobin weekly in patients on ESA who are not stable. Parathyroid hormone (PTH) should be monitored every 3 months, and other nutritional parameters should be monitored as needed.
[b]These measurements should be performed routinely in all patients/clients.
Source: Data are from reference 3.

DOCUMENTATION OF NUTRITION CARE

Documentation of nutrition care in the patient's/client's medical record is the primary way of communicating the nutrition goals and expected outcomes to the health care team. The documentation should be complete, concise, and in the format and style that is determined by facility or practice policy.

There are many different charting formats that can be used. Within the NCPM, a documentation model that follows the four steps of the NCP has been developed, using the ADIME (assessment, diagnosis, intervention, and monitoring and evaluation) format. If an electronic health record is being used, building standardized language into the health record will facilitate data collection and lead to a standardized nutrition data set. In 2009 the American Dietetic Association (now the Academy of Nutrition and Dietetics) published a white paper to address the need for a nutrition data set. This paper outlines the nutrition data-set elements needed in an electronic medical record: height and weight, body mass index, waist circumference, blood pressure, fasting lipoprotein profile, C-reactive protein, serum albumin, lifestyle habits assessment, level of physical fitness, and referral to the RD (56). Key elements to consider when charting each of the NCP steps can be found in Box 6.3 (23).

Box 6.3   Key Nutrition Care Process (NCP)–Related Charting Elements for Medical Records

Nutrition Assessment
- Date and time of assessment.
- Pertinent data collected and comparisons with standards (eg, food and nutrition history, biochemical data, anthropometric measurements, client history, medical nutrition therapy use, and supplement use).
- Patient's/client's readiness to learn, food and nutrition-related knowledge, and potential for change.
- Physical activity history and goals.
- Reason for discontinuation of nutrition therapy, if appropriate.

(continued)

Box 6.3   Key Nutrition Care Process (NCP)–Related Charting Elements for Medical Records (continued)

Nutrition Diagnosis
- Date and time.
- Concise written statement of nutrition diagnosis/diagnoses written in the PES (problem, etiology, signs and symptoms) format.
- If there is no existing nutrition problem, state "no nutrition diagnosis at this time."

Nutrition Intervention
- Date and time.
- Specific treatment goals and expected outcomes.
- Recommended nutrition prescription and individualized nutrition intervention.
- Any adjustments to plan and justification.
- Patient's/client's attitude regarding recommendations.
- Changes in patient's/client's attitude regarding recommendations.
- Changes in patient's/client's level of understanding and food-related behaviors.
- Referrals made and resources used.
- Any other information relevant to providing care and monitoring progress over time.
- Plans for follow-up and frequency.

Nutrition Monitoring and Evaluation
- Date and time.
- Specific nutrition outcome indicators and results relevant to the nutrition diagnosis and intervention plans and goals, compared with previous status or reference goals.
- Progress toward nutrition intervention goals.
- Factors facilitating or hindering progress.
- Other positive or negative outcomes.
- Future plans for nutrition care, monitoring, and follow-up or discharge.

Source: Adapted with permission from reference 23: Franz MJ, Boucher JL, Pereira RF. *ADA Pocket Guide to Lipid Disorders, Hypertension, Diabetes, and Weight Management.* Chicago, IL: American Dietetic Association; 2011.

CASE STUDY—NCP STEP 4:
NUTRITION MONITORING AND EVALUATION

Full nutrition assessment data for this case study of a 56-year-old Cambodian woman with ESRD are presented at the end of Chapter 2; nutrition diagnoses are listed at the end of Chapter 3; and the nutrition interventions are described at the ends of Chapters 4 and 5. In this final installment, outcome indicators are described using the standardized language of the NCP; criteria to evaluate outcomes are also listed (see Table 6.1).

Table 6.1   Case Study Outcome Indicators

Outcome Indicator	Criteria
Food and Nutrition-Related History	
Protein intake (FH 1.5.2)	Patient can explain how peritonitis affects protein needs; will identify foods to add 10–14 g protein per day.
Vitamin intake (FH 1.6.1)	Patient takes renal-specific multivitamin; does not take added vitamin C.
Mineral intake—Sodium (FH 1.6.2.7)	Patient uses less fish sauce (nouc mam) and less of other high-sodium sauces.
Mineral intake—Phosphorus (FH 1.6.2.6)	Patient decreases use of cola to treat nausea
Beliefs and attitudes (FH 4.2)	Patient understands the severity of risk to her health.

(continued)

Table 6.1   Case Study Outcome Indicators (continued)

Outcome Indicator	Criteria
Biochemical Data, Medical Tests, and Procedures	
Nutritional anemia profile (BD 1.10)	Team will evaluate iron stores and adjust treatment as appropriate.
Electrolyte and renal profile (BD 1.2)	Patient can explain at least one of the monthly tests and how her diet can be adjusted in context of results.
Anthropometric Measurements	
Weight change (AD 1.1.4)	Gradual decrease in patient's BMI to less than 30.
Nutrition-Focused Physical Findings	
Extremities, muscles, bones (PD 1.1.4) Head and eyes (PD 1.1.6)	Patient has less edema in legs and in face.

Appendix

Common Renal-Specific Vitamins

The products listed in this appendix are not all-inclusive of renal vitamins, and contents are subject to change. Check manufacturer Web sites and product labeling for up-to-date information.

Box A.1   Prescription Products

DexFol
Folic acid: 5 mg; thiamin (B-1): 1.5 mg; riboflavin (B-2): 1.5 mg; niacin (B-3): 20 mg; pantothenic acid (B-5): 10 mg; pyridoxine (B-6): 50 mg; cobalamin (B-12): 1,000 mcg; biotin: 300 mcg; vitamin C: 60 mg; vitamin D3: 0 IU; vitamin E: 0 IU; zinc: 0 mg; copper: 0 mg; selenium: 0 mcg

---

Dialyvite Rx
Folic acid: 1 mg; thiamin (B-1): 1.5 mg; riboflavin (B-2): 1.7 mg; niacin (B-3): 20 mg; pantothenic acid (B-5): 10 mg; pyridoxine (B-6): 10 mg; cobalamin (B-12): 6 mcg; biotin: 300 mcg; vitamin C: 100 mg; vitamin D3: 0 IU; vitamin E: 0 IU; zinc: 0 mg; copper: 0 mg; selenium: 0 mcg

---

Dialyvite w/Zinc Rx
Folic acid: 1 mg; thiamin (B-1): 1.5 mg; riboflavin (B-2): 1.7 mg; niacin (B-3): 20 mg; pantothenic acid (B-5): 10 mg; pyridoxine (B-6): 10 mg; cobalamin (B-12): 6 mcg; biotin: 300 mcg; vitamin C: 100 mg; vitamin D3: 0 IU; vitamin E: 0 IU; zinc: 50 mg; copper: 0 mg; selenium: 0 mcg

(continued)

Box A.1   Prescription Products (continued)

Dialyvite 3000
Folic acid: 3 mg; thiamin (B-1): 1.5 mg; riboflavin (B-2):
1.7 mg; niacin (B-3): 20 mg; pantothenic acid (B-5): 10 mg;
pyridoxine (B-6): 25 mg; cobalamin (B-12): 1,000 mcg; biotin:
300 mcg; vitamin C: 100 mg; vitamin D3: 0 IU; vitamin E:
30 IU; zinc: 15 mg; copper: 0 mg; selenium: 70 mcg

Dialyvite 5000
Folic acid: 5 mg; thiamin (B-1): 1.5 mg; riboflavin (B-2):
1.7 mg; niacin (B-3): 20 mg; pantothenic acid (B-5): 10 mg;
pyridoxine (B-6): 50 mg; cobalamin (B-12): 2,000 mcg; biotin:
300 mcg; vitamin C: 100 mg; vitamin D3: 0 IU; vitamin E:
30 IU; zinc: 25 mg; copper: 0 mg; selenium: 70 mcg

Dialyvite Supreme D Rx
Folic acid: 3 mg; thiamin (B-1): 1.5 mg; riboflavin (B-2):
1.7 mg; niacin (B-3): 20 mg; pantothenic acid (B-5): 10 mg;
pyridoxine (B-6): 25 mg; cobalamin (B-12): 1,000 mcg; biotin:
300 mcg; vitamin C: 100 mg; vitamin D3: 2,000 IU; vitamin E:
30 IU; zinc: 15 mg; copper: 0 mg; selenium: 70 mcg

Diatx Zn
Folic acid: 5 mg; thiamin (B-1): 1.5 mg; riboflavin (B-2):
1.7 mg; niacin (B-3): 20 mg; pantothenic acid (B-5): 10 mg;
pyridoxine (B-6): 50 mg; cobalamin (B-12): 2,000 mcg; biotin: 300 mcg; vitamin C: 60 mg; vitamin D3: 0 IU; vitamin E:
0 IU; zinc: 25 mg; copper: 1.5 mg; selenium: 0 mcg

Folbee Plus
Folic acid: 5 mg; thiamin (B-1): 1.5 mg; riboflavin (B-2):
1.7 mg; niacin (B-3): 20 mg; pantothenic acid (B-5): 10 mg;
pyridoxine (B-6): 50 mg; cobalamin (B-12): 1,000 mcg; biotin: 300 mcg; vitamin C: 60 mg; vitamin D3: 0 IU; vitamin E:
0 IU; zinc: 0 mg; copper: 0 mg; selenium: 0 mcg

(continued)

Box A.1   Prescription Products (continued)

Folbee Plus CZ
Folic acid: 5 mg; thiamin (B-1): 1.5 mg; riboflavin (B-2): 1.7 mg; niacin (B-3): 20 mg; pantothenic acid (B-5): 10 mg; pyridoxine (B-6): 50 mg; cobalamin (B-12): 2,000 mcg; biotin: 300 mcg; vitamin C: 60 mg; vitamin D3: 0 IU; vitamin E: 0 IU; zinc: 25 mg; copper: 1.5 mg; selenium: 0 mcg

Nephrocap
Folic acid: 1 mg; thiamin (B-1): 1.5 mg; riboflavin (B-2): 1.7 mg; niacin (B-3): 20 mg; pantothenic acid (B-5): 5 mg; pyridoxine (B-6): 10 mg; cobalamin (B-12): 6 mcg; biotin: 300 mcg; vitamin C: 100 mg; vitamin D3: 0 IU; vitamin E: 0 IU; zinc: 0 mg; copper: 0 mg; selenium: 0 mcg

Nephronex Caps
Folic acid: 1 mg; thiamin (B-1): 1.5 mg; riboflavin (B-2): 1.7 mg; niacin (B-3): 20 mg; pantothenic acid (B-5): 10 mg; pyridoxine (B-6): 10 mg; cobalamin (B-12): 10 mcg; biotin: 150 mcg; vitamin C: 60 mg; vitamin D3: 0 IU; vitamin E: 0 IU; zinc: 0 mg; copper: 0 mg; selenium: 0 mcg

Nephro-Vite Rx
Folic acid: 1 mg; thiamin (B-1): 1.5 mg; riboflavin (B-2): 1.7 mg; niacin (B-3): 20 mg; pantothenic acid (B-5): 10 mg; pyridoxine (B-6): 10 mg; cobalamin (B-12): 6 mcg; biotin: 300 mcg; vitamin C: 60 mg; vitamin D3: 0 IU; vitamin E: 0 IU; zinc: 0 mg; copper: 0 mg; selenium: 0 mcg

Renax
Folic acid: 2.5 mg; thiamin (B-1): 3 mg; riboflavin (B-2): 2 mg; niacin (B-3): 20 mg; pantothenic acid (B-5): 10 mg; pyridoxine (B-6): 15 mg; cobalamin (B-12): 12 mcg; biotin: 300 mcg; vitamin C: 50 mg; vitamin D3: 0 IU; vitamin E: 35 IU; zinc: 20 mg; copper: 0 mg; selenium: 70 mcg

(continued)

Box A.1 **Prescription Products** (continued)

Renax 5.5

Folic acid: 5.5 mg; thiamin (B-1): 3 mg; riboflavin (B-2): 2 mg; niacin (B-3): 20 mg; pantothenic acid (B-5): 10 mg; pyridoxine (B-6): 30 mg; cobalamin (B-12): 1,000 mcg; biotin: 300 mcg; vitamin C: 100 mg; vitamin D3: 0 IU; vitamin E: 35 IU; zinc: 20 mg; copper: 0 mg; selenium: 70 mcg

---

Vital-D Rx

Folic acid: 1 mg; thiamin (B-1): 1.5 mg; riboflavin (B-2): 1.7 mg; niacin (B-3): 20 mg; pantothenic acid (B-5): 10 mg; pyridoxine (B-6): 10 mg; cobalamin (B-12): 6 mcg; biotin: 300 mcg; vitamin C: 60 mg; vitamin D3: 1,750 IU; vitamin E: 0 IU; zinc: 12.5 mg; copper: 0 mg; selenium: 0 mcg

---

Manufacturers: Dexfol: Rising Pharmaceuticals, Inc, Allendale, NJ, www .risingpharma.com; Dialyvite Rx, Dialyvite w/Zinc Rx, Dialyvite 3000, Dialyvite 5000, Dialyvite Supreme D Rx: Hillestad Pharmaceuticals USA Inc, Woodruff, WI, www.hillestadlabs.com; DiatxZn: Centrix Pharmaceuticals, Birmingham, AL 35242, www.cenrx.com; Folbee Plus and Folbee Plus CZ: Breckenridge Pharmaceuticals, Boca Raton, FL, www.golbeeplus.com; Nephrocap: Fleming Pharmaceuticals, Fenton, MO, www.flemingpharma .com; Nephronex Caps: Llorens Pharmaceuticals, Miami, FL, www.llorens pharm.com; Nephro-Vite Rx: Watson Pharmaceuticals, Morristown, NJ, www .watson.com; Renax and Renax 5.5: Everett Laboratories, West Orange, NJ, www.everettlabs.com; Vital-D Rx: Nephro-Tech, Shawnee Mission, KS, www.nephrotech.com.

Source: Data are from reference 35.

Box A.2   Over-the-Counter Products

Dialyvite 800
Folic acid: 0.8 mg; thiamin (B-1): 1.5 mg; riboflavin (B-2): 1.7 mg; niacin (B-3): 20 mg; pantothenic acid (B-5): 10 mg; pyridoxine (B-6): 10 mg; cobalamin (B-12): 6 mcg; biotin: 300 mcg; vitamin C: 60 mg; vitamin D3: 0 IU; vitamin E: 0 IU; zinc: 0 mg; copper: 0 mg; selenium: 0 mcg

---

Dialyvite 800 w/Iron
Folic acid: 0.8 mg; thiamin (B-1): 1.5 mg; riboflavin (B-2): 1.7 mg; niacin (B-3): 20 mg; pantothenic acid (B-5): 10 mg; pyridoxine (B-6): 10 mg; cobalamin (B-12): 6 mcg; biotin: 300 mcg; vitamin C: 60 mg; vitamin D3: 0 IU; vitamin E: 0 IU; zinc: 0 mg; copper: 0 mg; selenium: 0 mcg

---

Dialyvite 800 w/Zinc
Folic acid: 0.8 mg; thiamin (B-1): 1.5 mg; riboflavin (B-2): 1.7 mg; niacin (B-3): 20 mg; pantothenic acid (B-5): 10 mg; pyridoxine (B-6): 10 mg; cobalamin (B-12): 6 mcg; biotin: 300 mcg; vitamin C: 60 mg; vitamin D3: 0 IU; vitamin E: 0 IU; zinc: 50 mg; copper: 0 mg; selenium: 0 mcg

---

Dialyvite 800 w/Zinc 15
Folic acid: 0.8 mg; thiamin (B-1): 1.5 mg; riboflavin (B-2): 1.7 mg; niacin (B-3): 20 mg; pantothenic acid (B-5): 10 mg; pyridoxine (B-6): 10 mg; cobalamin (B-12): 6 mcg; biotin: 300 mcg; vitamin C: 60 mg; vitamin D3: 0 IU; vitamin E: 0 IU; zinc: 15 mg; copper: 0 mg; selenium: 0 mcg

---

Dialyvite Ultra D
Folic acid: 0.8 mg; thiamin (B-1): 1.5 mg; riboflavin (B-2): 1.7 mg; niacin (B-3): 20 mg; pantothenic acid (B-5): 10 mg; pyridoxine (B-6): 10 mg; cobalamin (B-12): 6 mcg; biotin: 300 mcg; vitamin C: 60 mg; vitamin D3: 2,000 IU; vitamin E: 30 IU; zinc: 15 mg; copper: 0 mg; selenium: 70 mcg

(continued)

Box A.2   Over-the-Counter Products (continued)

Nephronex Liquid
Folic acid: 0.9 mg; thiamin (B-1): 1.5 mg; riboflavin (B-2): 1.7 mg; niacin (B-3): 20 mg; pantothenic acid (B-5): 10 mg; pyridoxine (B-6): 10 mg; cobalamin (B-12): 10 mcg; biotin: 300 mcg; vitamin C: 60 mg; vitamin D3: 0 IU; vitamin E: 0 IU; zinc: 0 mg; copper: 0 mg; selenium: 0 mcg

Nephro-Vite
Folic acid: 0.8 mg; thiamin (B-1): 1.5 mg; riboflavin (B-2): 1.7 mg; niacin (B-3): 20 mg; pantothenic acid (B-5): 10 mg; pyridoxine (B-6): 10 mg; cobalamin (B-12): 6 mcg; biotin: 300 mcg; vitamin C: 60 mg; vitamin D3: 0 IU; vitamin E: 0 IU; zinc: 0 mg; copper: 0 mg; selenium: 0 mcg

ProRenal QD
Folic acid: 0.8 mg; thiamin (B-1): 1.5 mg; riboflavin (B-2): 2.0 mg; niacin (B-3): 20 mg; pantothenic acid (B-5): 5 mg; pyridoxine (B-6): 5 mg; cobalamin (B-12): 2.4 mcg; biotin: 300 mcg; vitamin C: 60 mg; vitamin D3: 800 IU; vitamin E: 10 IU; zinc: 8 mg; copper: 0.9 mg; selenium: 55 mcg

Renal Factor
Folic acid: 0.8 mg; thiamin (B-1): 1.5 mg; riboflavin (B-2): 1.7 mg; niacin (B-3): 20 mg; pantothenic acid (B-5): 10 mg; pyridoxine (B-6): 10 mg; cobalamin (B-12): 6 mcg; biotin: 300 mcg; vitamin C: 60 mg; vitamin D3: 0 IU; vitamin E: 0 IU; zinc: 0 mg; copper: 0 mg; selenium: 0 mcg

Renal Tab II
Folic acid: 1 mg; thiamin (B-1): 1.5 mg; riboflavin (B-2): 1.7 mg; niacin (B-3): 20 mg; pantothenic acid (B-5): 10 mg; pyridoxine (B-6): 10 mg; cobalamin (B-12): 6 mcg; biotin: 300 mcg; vitamin C: 60 mg; vitamin D3: 0 IU; vitamin E: 0 IU; zinc: 0 mg; copper: 0 mg; selenium: 0 mcg

(continued)

Box A.2   Over-the-Counter Products (continued)

Renal Tab Zn

Folic acid: 1 mg; thiamin (B-1): 1.5 mg; riboflavin (B-2):
1.7 mg; niacin (B-3): 20 mg; pantothenic acid (B-5): 10 mg;
pyridoxine (B-6): 10 mg; cobalamin (B-12): 6 mcg; biotin:
300 mcg; vitamin C: 60 mg; vitamin D3: 0 IU; vitamin E:
0 IU; zinc: 15 mg; copper: 0 mg; selenium: 0 mcg

Renal Tab Zn + D

Folic acid: 1 mg; thiamin (B-1): 1.5 mg; riboflavin (B-2):
1.7 mg; niacin (B-3): 20 mg; pantothenic acid (B-5): 10 mg;
pyridoxine (B-6): 10 mg; cobalamin (B-12): 6 mcg; biotin:
300 mcg; vitamin C: 60 mg; vitamin D3: 1,000 IU; vitamin E:
0 IU; zinc: 15 mg; copper: 0 mg; selenium: 0 mcg

RenaPlex

Folic acid: 0.8 mg; thiamin (B-1): 1.5 mg; riboflavin (B-2):
1.7 mg; niacin (B-3): 20 mg; pantothenic acid (B-5): 10 mg;
pyridoxine (B-6): 10 mg; cobalamin (B-12): 6 mcg; biotin:
300 mcg; vitamin C: 60 mg; vitamin D3: 0 IU; vitamin E:
0 IU; zinc: 12.5 mg; copper: 0 mg; selenium: 0 mcg

RenaVit

Folic acid: 0.8 mg; thiamin (B-1): 1.5 mg; riboflavin (B-2):
1.7 mg; niacin (B-3): 20 mg; pantothenic acid (B-5): 10 mg;
pyridoxine (B-6): 10 mg; cobalamin (B-12): 6 mcg; biotin:
300 mcg; vitamin C: 60 mg; vitamin D3: 0 IU; vitamin E:
0 IU; zinc: 0 mg; copper: 0 mg; selenium: 0 mcg

Manufacturers: Dialyvite 800, Dialyvite 800 w/Iron, Dialyvite 800 w/Zinc,
Dialyvite 800 w/Zinc 15, and Dialyvite Ultra D: Hillestad Pharmaceuticals
USA Inc, Woodruff, WI, www.hillestadlabs.com; RenaPlex: Nephro-Tech,
Shawnee Mission, KS, www.nephrotech.com; Nephronex Liquid: Llorens
Pharmaceuticals, Miami, FL, www.llorenspharm.com; Nephro-Vite:
Watson Pharmaceuticals, Morristown, NJ, www.watson.com; Renal Factor:
Healthy Factor, Arbor Vitae, WI; RenalTab II, RenalTab Zn, and RenalTab
Zn + D: Renalab Inc, Templeton, CA 93465, www.renalabs.com; ProRenal
QD: Nephroceuticals, Miamisburg, OH, www.myprorenal.com; RenaVit:
Integrative Therapeutics, Green Bay, WI, www.integrativeinc.com.
Source: Data are from reference 35.

References

1. Academy of Nutrition and Dietetics. *International Dietetics & Nutrition Terminology (IDNT) Reference Manual: Standardized Language for the Nutrition Care Process*, 4th ed. Chicago, IL: Academy of Nutrition and Dietetics; 2013.

2. Academy of Nutrition and Dietetics. Evidence Analysis Library. Evidence-Based Nutrition Practice Guidelines for Chronic Kidney Disease. www.adaevidencelibrary.com/topic.cfm?cat=3929.

3. National Kidney Foundation. Clinical practice guidelines for nutrition in chronic renal failure. K/DOQI, National Kidney Foundation. *Am J Kidney Dis.* 2000;35(6)(suppl 2)S1–S140. www.kidney.org/professionals/KDOQI/guidelines_updates/doqi_nut.html.

4. National Kidney Foundation. KDOQI clinical practice guidelines and clinical practice recommendations for diabetes and chronic kidney disease. *Am J Kidney Dis.* 2007;49(2 suppl 2):S1–S180. www.kidney.org/professionals/KDOQI/guideline_diabetes.

5. National Kidney Foundation. KDOQI clinical practice guideline for diabetes and CKD: 2012 update. *Am J Kidney Dis.* 2012;60(5):850–886. www.kidney.org/professionals/KDOQI/guidelines_diabetesUp/diabetes-ckd-update-2012.pdf.

6. National Kidney Foundation. KDOQI clinical practice guidelines for chronic kidney disease: evaluation, classification, and stratification. *Am J Kidney Dis.* 2002;39(suppl 1):S1–S266. www.kidney.org/professionals/KDOQI/guidelines_ckd/p4_class_g1.htm.

7. National Kidney Foundation. KDOQI clinical practice guidelines and clinical practice recommendations for anemia in chronic kidney disease. *Am J Kidney Dis.* 2006;47(5 suppl 3):S11–S145. www.kidney.org/professionals/KDOQI/guidelines_anemia/index.htm.

8. National Kidney Foundation. KDOQI clinical practice guidelines for hypertension and antihypertensive agents in chronic kidney disease. *Am J Kidney Dis.* 2004;41(5 suppl 1):S1–S290.

www.kidney.org/professionals/KDOQI/guidelines_bp/index
.htm.

9. National Kidney Foundation. KDOQI clinical practice guidelines for managing dyslipidemias in chronic kidney disease. *Am
   J Kidney Dis.* 2003;41(suppl 3):S1–S92. www.kidney.org/pro
   fessionals/KDOQI/guidelines_lipids/toc.htm.

10. Kidney Disease: Improving Global Outcomes (KDIGO) CKD-
    MBD Work Group. KDIGO clinical practice guidelines for the
    diagnosis, evaluation, prevention, and treatment of chronic
    kidney disease-mineral and bone disorder (CKD-MBD). *Kid-
    ney Int.* 2009; 76 (suppl 113):S1–S130. www.kdigo.org/clini
    cal_practice_guidelines/kdigo_guideline_for_ckd-mbd.php.

11. KDIGO. KDIGO 2012 clinical practice guideline for the evalua-
    tion and management of chronic kidney disease. *Kidney Int Suppl.*
    2013;3(1):26–32. www.kdigo.org/clinical_practice_guidelines
    /pdf/CKD/KDIGO_2012_CKD_GL.pdf.

12. Centers for Medicare & Medicaid Services. Department of
    Health and Human Services. Conditions for Coverage for End-
    Stage Renal Disease Facilities. *Federal Register.* April 15, 2008.
    73(73):20370–20484. www.cms.hhs.gov/center/esrd.asp.

13. Centers for Medicare & Medicaid Services. Department of
    Health and Human Services. *The Guide to Medicare Preven-
    tive Services.* 4th ed. March 2011: 127–128. www.cms.gov
    /Outreach-and-Education/Medicare-Learning-Network-MLN
    /MLNProducts/downloads/mps_guide_web-061305.pdf.

14. Brown RO, Comphor C. A.S.P.E.N. clinical guidelines: nutri-
    tion support in adult acute and chronic renal failure. *JPEN J
    Parenter Enteral Nutr.* 2010;34:366–377. www.nutritioncare
    .org/Professional_Resources/Guidelines_and_Standards/Guide
    lines/2010_Nutrition_Support_in_Adult_Acute_and_Chronic
    _Renal_Failure.

15. Martindale RG, McClave SA, Vanek VW, McCarthy M, Rob-
    erts P, Taylor B, Ochoa JB, Neopolitano L, Cresci G. Guidelines
    for the provision and assessment of nutrition support therapy
    in the adult critically ill patient: Society of Critical Care Medi-
    cine and American Society for Parenteral and Enteral Nutrition:
    executive summary. *Crit Care Med.* 2009;37:1757–1761.

16. Fouque D, Vennegoor M, Wee PT, Wanner C, Basci A, Canaud
    B, Haage P, Konner K, Kooman J, Martin-Malo A, Pedrini L,

Pizzarelli F, Tattersal J, Tordoir J, Vanholder R. EBPG guideline on nutrition. *Nephrol Dial Transplant.* 2007;22: ii45–ii87.

17. Chadban S, Chan M, Fry K, Patwardhan A, Ryan C, Trevillian P, Westgarth F. CARI Transplant Guidelines: Nutrition in Kidney Transplant Recipients. *Nephrology.* 2010;15:S35–S71.

18. Academy of Nutrition and Dietetics. Medical Nutrition Therapy. www.eatright.org/HealthProfessionals/content.aspx?id=6877.

19. Academy of Nutrition and Dietetics Evidence Analysis Library. Flowchart of encounters 2011. *Chronic Kidney Disease Toolkit.* Chicago, IL: Academy of Nutrition and Dietetics (in press).

20. Centers for Medicare & Medicaid Services. Department of Health and Human Services. Survey & certification: guidance to laws & regulations—dialysis. ESRD program interpretive guidance. www.cms.gov/GuidanceforLawsAndRegulations/05_Dialysis.asp.

21. McCarthy M, Asbell D. A Renal Nutrition Forum series with practice-based examples of the Nutrition Care Process (NCP): where does nutrition diagnosis fit in the new Conditions for Coverage? *Renal Nutrition Forum.* 2009;28(2):20–23.

22. Belibi FA, Wallace DP, Yamaguchi T, Christensen M, Reif G, Grantham JJ. The effect of caffeine on renal epithelial cells from patients with autosomal dominant polycystic kidney disease. *J Am Soc Nephrol.* 2002;13:2723–2729.

23. Franz MJ, Boucher JL, Pereira RF. *ADA Pocket Guide to Lipid Disorders, Hypertension, Diabetes, and Weight Management.* Chicago, IL: American Dietetic Association; 2011.

24. McCann L, ed. *Pocket Guide to Nutrition Assessment of the Patient with Chronic Kidney Disease,* 4th ed. New York, NY: National Kidney Foundation; 2009.

25. McPartland J, Pomposelli JJ. Update on immunosuppressive drugs used in solid-organ transplantation and their nutrition implications. *Nutr Clin Pract.* 2007;22:467–473.

26. World Health Organization (WHO). Global database on body mass index. BMI classification. http://apps.who.int/bmi/index.jsp?introPage=intro_3.html.

27. Frisancho AR. New standards of weight and body composition by frame size and height for assessment of nutritional status of adults and the elderly. *Am J Clin Nutr.* 1984;40:808-819.

28. Wiggins KL. *Guidelines for Nutrition Care of Renal Patients.* Chicago, IL: American Dietetic Association; 2001.

29. Third Report of the National Cholesterol Education Program (NCEP) Expert Panel on Detection, Evaluation, and Treatment of High Blood Cholesterol in Adults (Adult Treatment Panel III). Bethesda, MD: National Cholesterol Education Program, National Heart, Lung, and Blood Institute, and National Institutes of Health; 2001. NIH Publication No. 01-3670. www.nhlbi .nih.gov/guidelines/cholesterol/atp3full.pdf.

30. National Kidney Foundation. KDOQI clinical practice guidelines for bone metabolism and disease in chronic kidney disease. *Am J Kidney Dis.* 2003;42(suppl 3):S1-S201.

31. Steiber A, Kopple J. Vitamin status and needs for people with stages 3-5 Chronic Kidney Disease. *J Ren Nutr.* 2011;21:355–368.

32. Pronsky ZM, Crowe JP. *Food and Medication Interactions.* 16th ed. Birchrunville, PA: Food-Medication Interactions; 2010.

33. Kidney Disease: Improving Global Outcomes (KDIGO) Anemia Work Group. KDIGO clinical practice guideline for anemia in chronic kidney disease. *Kidney Int Suppl.* 2012;2(4):283–287. www.kdigo.org/clinical_practice_guidelines/anemia.php.

34. Matarese LE, Steiger E, Seidner DL, McAdams MP, DeChicco RS, Speerhas R, Curtas S, Katz D, Jeris de Burgoa L. *The Cleveland Clinic Foundation Nutrition Support Handbook.* Cleveland, OH: The Cleveland Clinic Foundation; 1997.

35. Byham-Gray L, Wiesen K, Stover J. *A Clinical Guide to Nutrition Care in Kidney Disease,* 2nd ed. Chicago, IL: The Academy of Nutrition and Dietetics; 2013.

36. Krediet RT. European Best Practice Guideline on peritoneal dialysis: nutrition in peritoneal dialysis. *Nephrol Dial Transplant.* 2005;20(9): ix28–ix33.

37. Ishibe S, Peixoto AJ. Methods of assessment of volume status and intercompartmental fluid shifts in hemodialysis patients: implications in clinical practice. *Semin Dial.* 2004;17:37–43.

38. Sinha AD, Light RP, Agarwal R. Relative plasma volume monitoring during hemodialysis aids the assessment of dry weight. *Hypertension.* 2010;55:305–311.

39. Byham-Gray L, Wiesen K. *A Clinical Guide to Nutrition Care in Kidney Disease*. Chicago, IL: American Dietetic Association; 2004.

40. Davita. A brief overview of home hemodialysis. www.davita
.com/treatment-options/home-hemodialysis/what-is-home
-hemodialysis-/a-brief-overview-of-home-hemodialysis/t/5578.

41. National Kidney Center. Home hemodialysis. www.national
kidneycenter.org/treatment-options/kidney-dialysis/home
-hemodialysis/?gclid=CJTmj6KB-rQCFemiPAod3SQ.

42. Davita. Nocturnal in-center hemodialysis. www.davita.com
/treatment-options/in-center-nocturnal-dialysis/what-is-noc
turnal-dialysis/in-center-nocturnal-dialysis-and-your-kidney
-diet/t/5607.

43. Fresenius Medical Care. In-center dialysis. www.ultracare-dial-
ysis.com/Treatment/InCenterDialysis.aspx.

44. Blue LS. Adult kidney transplantation. In: Hasse JM, Blue LS.
Comprehensive Guide to Transplant Nutrition. Chicago, IL:
American Dietetic Association; 2002:45–56.

45. American Dietetic Association. *National Renal Diet: Professional Guide.* 2nd ed. Chicago, IL: American Dietetic Association; 2002.

46. Wiggins KL, Harvey KS. A review of guidelines for nutrition
care of renal patients. *J Ren Nutr.* 2002;12(3):190–196.

47. National Kidney Foundation. KDOQI clinical practice guidelines for cardiovascular disease in dialysis patients. *Am J Kidney
Dis.* 2005;45(4 suppl 3):S1-S153. www.kidney.org/profession
als/KDOQI/guidelines_cvd/index.htm.

48. Obayashi PAC. Food safety for the solid organ transplant patient:
preventing foodborne illness while on chronic immunosuppressive drugs. *Nutr Clin Pract.* 2012;27:758–766.

49. VanWormer JJ, Boucher JL. The 5 A's: behavior change counseling in the context of brief clinical encounters. *On the Cutting
Edge.* 2003;24(4):24–26.

50. VanWormer JJ, Boucher JL. Motivational interviewing and diabetes education: fostering commitment to change. *On the Cutting Edge.* 2003;24(4):14–16.

51. VanWormer JJ, Boucher JL. Motivational interviewing and
diet modification: a review of the evidence. *Diabetes Educ.*
2004;30:404–419.

52. Prochaska JO, Velicer WF. The transtheoretical model of health
behavior changes. *Am J Health Promot.* 1997;12:38–48.

53. Gehling E. Changing us or changing them? *Newsflash* (newsletter of the Diabetes Care and Education Dietetic Practice Group). Chicago, IL: American Dietetic Association. 1999;29:31–33.

54. Artinian NT, Fletcher GF, Mozaffarian D, Kris-Etherton P, Van Horn L, Lichtenstein AH, Kumanyika S, Kraus WE, Fleg JL, Redeker NS, Meininger JC, Banks J, Stuart-Shor EM, Fletcher BJ, Miller TD, Hughes S, Braun LT, Kopin LA, Berra K, Hayman LL, Ewing LJ, Ades PA, Durstine JL, Houston-Miller N, Burke LE. American Heart Association Prevention Committee of the Council on Cardiovascular Nursing. Interventions to promote physical activity and dietary lifestyle changes for cardiovascular risk factor reduction in adults: a scientific statement from the American Heart Association. *Circulation.* 2010;122:406–441.

55. Klein S, Burke LE, Gray GA, Glair S, Allison DB, Pi-Sunyer X, Hong Y, Ecker RH. Clinical implications of obesity with specific focus on cardiovascular disease: a statement for professionals from the American Heart Association Council on Nutrition, Physical Activity, and Metabolism. *Circulation.* 2004;110:2952–2967.

56. Peregrin T. Personal and electronic health records: sharing nutrition information across the health care community. *J Am Diet Assoc.* 2009;109:1988–1991.

Index

Page number followed by *b* signifies a box; *t* signifies a table.